The Vasectomy Book

The Vasectomy Book

A Complete Guide to Decision Making

MARC GOLDSTEIN, M.D.

AND MICHAEL FELDBERG, Ph.D.

Foreword by C. Wayne Bardin, M.D.
Vice President of the Population Council and
Director, Center for Biomedical Research

J. P. TARCHER, INC.
Los Angeles
Distributed by Houghton Mifflin Company
Boston

J. P. Tarcher, Inc.
9110 Sunset Blvd.
Los Angeles, CA 90069

Library of Congress Cataloging in Publication Data

Goldstein, Marc.
    The vasectomy book.

    Includes index.
    1. Vasectomy.   2. Vasectomy—Decision making.
3. Vasovasostomy.   4. Contraceptives.   I. Feldberg,
Michael.   II. Title.
RD585.5.G64   613.9'42   81-85210
ISBN 0-87477-207-9   AACR2

Manufactured in the United States of America
S 10 9 8 7 6 5 4 3 2 1

First Edition

For Jody and Ruth

Contents

Foreword

As recently as thirty years ago, medical students were taught that vasectomy could be used for birth control but that it should be used with reservation because there were severe emotional and perhaps physical complications associated with the procedure. An examination of the history of vasectomy gives some insight into the reasons for this apprehension. In the late 1800s, vasectomies were performed for a variety of reasons including impotence, infection, rejuvenation of the aged, and improvement of health. In the early decades of the nineteenth century, vasectomy was recommended for the poor and for criminals so that their children would not become wards of the state. By the 1950s, these uses of vasectomy had been discredited and the association of sterilization with the atrocities of World War II made sterilization unsavory for any purpose in the eyes of many individuals. In addition, new contraceptives for females were being developed which offered the hope of highly effective, convenient contraception capable of solving the world's population problem.

Many factors have resulted in a change in perception

of vasectomy through the 1960s and '70s. It is now considered a highly desirable form of contraception for many couples. The reasons for this change in outlook, along with insights on why vasectomy is now recommended only for contraceptive purposes, are clearly presented in the first portion of *The Vasectomy Book*.

This is a highly personal book, recommended for individuals who are considering the procedure and who want to decide whether this form of birth control is suitable for them. To help in this goal, Dr. Marc Goldstein and Michael Feldberg first present a detailed description of the male reproductive tract. A discussion of the structure and function of each organ is provided in sufficient detail to provide the reader with an overview of male sexuality and reproductive function. With this as a background, what vasectomy accomplishes is, therefore, quite easy to understand. Having presented the anatomy of a vasectomy, the authors then proceed with considerations of the psychological and emotional issues surrounding this procedure. A useful questionnaire is provided to help the reader understand the problems that can be associated with this form of birth control. This is a useful process, as it provides a self-counseling procedure that might be difficult to duplicate from a physician or other birth-planning practitioner.

The surgical procedure, recovery, and possible complications are reviewed in graphic detail. The questions covered include what will actually happen in the hospital, how long recovery will take, why contraception must be continued immediately following the surgical procedure, why postoperative sperm counts are necessary, and many others. The authors even point out the embarrassment associated with the visit to the doctor's office for the first postoperative sperm count.

When any procedure is recommended for family planning, the major and overriding concern is safety. Recent observations in monkeys have raised questions as to whether vasectomy might increase the risk of heart attack in some men. These concerns are thoughtfully reviewed, and an up-to-date assessment of the risks of human vasectomy is presented. When issues of safety are raised, one is entitled to ask, "How safe?" and, "Safe as compared to what?" These questions are particularly pertinent, since no procedure or medication can ever be entirely free of risk. To address these issues, the authors briefly review the advantages and disadvantages of vasectomy as compared to other popular family planning methods, such as the pill, IUDs, and barrier methods.

In this book, Goldstein and Feldberg provide a thorough and lucid treatment of vasectomy from many points of view. All of the important issues are discussed in balance. The book should be useful not only for individuals who are considering vasectomy but for physicians and family planners who must counsel individuals about the advisability of permanent sterilization.

C. Wayne Bardin, M.D.
Vice President of the Population Council and
Director, Center for Biomedical Research

Preface

This book grows out of our personal experience: Marc Goldstein's as an andrologist and urologic microsurgeon, Michael Feldberg's as a researcher, vasectomy patient, and reversal patient. For several years, we have been aware of the critical need for an up-to-date, accurate, and objective book to help men, women, and couples weigh the benefits and risks of male sterilization. *The Vasectomy Book* is intended to meet that need.

The Vasectomy Book functions on three levels: as a guide to what is known about the medical and psychological effects of vasectomy and reversal; as an introduction to the actual experience of a vasectomy or reversal; and as a process for deciding if sterilization is the best form of birth control for you. When we use the term "you," we have women as well as men in mind. As the text will make clear, we believe that sterilization is a choice that couples should make together rather than as individuals. At the same time, *The Vasectomy Book* acknowledges that single men may also be interested in either vasectomy or reversal.

Knowledge in the fields of male reproductive medicine, contraception, and microsurgery is changing rapidly. Innovations in surgical techniques are reported regularly, and new findings about the long-term effects of contraceptives, vasectomy, and hormones appear monthly in medical and scientific journals. Sometimes, one set of findings contradicts another. As a result, the reader will find us using such terms as "possibly," "may," or "are believed to" rather than more definitive formulations. This practice reflects our attempt to take an objective and cautious, one might even say conservative, approach to our subject. We hope that the reader will bring the same degree of deliberateness to his or her considerations. While we have offered advice in regard to both vasectomy and vasectomy reversal, final decisions in the realm of birth control choices rest ultimately with each individual and couple.

Acknowledgments

Books such as this one are made possible because many individuals are willing to assist the authors in their efforts. The following names comprise but a partial list of those who offered advice, help, typing, editing, moral support, or encouragement through the many stages of *The Vasectomy Book.*

Nancy Alexander, Ph.D.
Reta Blake
Ellen Bresnick, M.S.W.
Joseph E. Davis, M.D.
Bunny Duhl, Ed.D.
Janice Gallagher
Catherine Gallaway
Betty Gonzales, R.N.
Patrick deGramont, Ph.D.
Hugo Hoogenboom, L.L.B.
Elaine Jenkins
Paul Levenson, Ph.D.
Katinka Matson
Richard Sherins, M.D.

Sherman J. Silber, M.D.
Irving Sivin, M.A.
Joseph Stock
Karl Stull
Rebecca Smith
E. Darracot Vaughan, Jr., M.D.
Keith Waterhouse, M.D.

We also wish to thank our colleagues at: The Population Council's Center for Biomedical Research; Rockefeller University; New York Hospital-Cornell Medical Center; and Boston University. Finally, we wish to extend a special note of gratitude to C. Wayne Bardin, M.D., Vice President of the Population Council and Director, Center for Biomedical Research, who has provided invaluable advice, support, and encouragement for this project.

Introduction

This year, half a million American men will undergo vasectomy. According to the Association for Voluntary Sterilization, approximately 7 million American men have been sterilized for contraceptive purposes, virtually all of them since 1970. Among American couples in which the female is thirty years or older, one in twelve uses vasectomy as their means of contraception. Measured in terms of cost, effectiveness, and safety, vasectomy is probably the best available method of permanent contraception.

This is not to say that vasectomy is beyond controversy or that the procedure is recommended for every male who considers having one. In recent years, medical researchers have raised a number of issues about vasectomy's physical safety, suggesting that the operation may have negative consequences for a man's heart, his circulatory system, his kidneys, or his immune and reproductive systems. Psychological researchers have pointed out that some men seem vulnerable to emotional difficulties after vasectomy, which can unleash hidden conflicts and raise unexpected stress in marital or love relationships.

The Vasectomy Book grows out of our conviction that there is no reliable source available to the general reader that can help him or her sort out the complex issues surrounding vasectomy. To date, nearly all the popular books and articles have presented unbalanced views of the subject. Advocates have been almost completely uncritical of the operation, while those who have raised questions about its side effects tend to be alarmist and cynical.* Recent newspaper and magazine reports on the potential dangers of vasectomy present data out of context in an effort to grab reader attention rather than promote reader understanding.

We believe that for men and women to make intelligent choices about the appropriateness and safety of vasectomy, they need two things: current, clear information and a method for evaluating each option and its consequences. This book is intended to provide readers with an accurate and objective assessment of what is known and what needs to be known about vasectomy. For us it is paramount that each reader make a wise and well-informed decision for or against vasectomy based on his, her, or their enlightened self-regard. While vasectomy is but one choice among several measures against unplanned conception, its permanence (like the permanence of tubal ligation) puts vasectomy in a special category of birth control. Its potential impact on a man's emotional state, his sense of identity, his relationship to his wife or lover and their future life together necessitates the most deliberate and thoughtful discussion of alternatives and likely outcomes before reaching a decision. *The Vasectomy Book* offers the

---

*For those interested in further reading on the subject, we have included a References section listing additional books and articles.

clear and accurate information needed for that discussion.

In Chapter 1, we present the historical background of the operation, including its misuse for purposes other than effective, permanent birth control. By describing its past, we hope to distinguish the appropriate from inappropriate uses of vasectomy and to dispel a few myths. In Chapter 2, we take a detailed look at how the male reproductive system works and how vasectomy affects its functioning. Chapter 3 provides a method for men and couples to assess whether they are ready to adopt permanent contraception and whether the male or female is the more appropriate partner for sterilization.

These first three chapters will help you decide it you are at the right time and place in your life for considering vasectomy. The rest of the book gathers the information you need in order to determine which is the best method of birth control for you.

Chapter 4 previews what to expect from the experience of the vasectomy procedure, including how it will probably feel, and provides advice on taking care of yourself for the first few days after the operation. The potential for subsequent emotional problems is the topic of Chapter 5, which profiles individuals who have had difficulty making a psychological adjustment to sterilization. To help you evaluate the potential for any other long-term problems, Chapter 6 outlines all the known and suspected medical risks. Chapter 7 weighs the advantages and disadvantages of vasectomy against those of other methods of contraception widely available for both men and women.

This book also introduces a revolutionary microsurgical technique for reversing vasectomies in men who, for any number of good reasons, have reconsidered their original decision. Chapter 8 explains in detail how vasectomy reversal works, how you can find a physician to perform one, and what you can expect to experience in the days and weeks before and after a vasectomy reversal. Chapter 9 addresses vasectomy reversal as a decision, placing it in the context of a man's feelings about himself, his masculinity, and his marriage or love relationship. It also suggests methods for dealing with potential reversal failure.

In the final chapter, we explore the future of male birth control. The development of new testosterone-based drugs, such as Depo-Provera, and mechanical valves that can be implanted in the vas deferens offer the possibility of effective but nonpermanent male contraception. We conclude with an assessment of the long-range prospects for each of these alternatives.

1
A History
of Vasectomy

Vasectomy is nothing more than the surgical interruption of the two tubes that carry a man's sperm from his testicles to his ejaculatory ducts, where the sperm are stored before departing his body during orgasm. Since sperm can no longer leave a man's body after vasectomy, he can no longer make a woman pregnant. Thus, vasectomy is simply an effective, inexpensive, easy-to-perform method of contraception.*

In the past, vasectomy has been thought to have almost magical powers to effect great changes, both in an individual man and in society. Early vasectomy advocates claimed that the operation could rejuvenate a man, making him younger physically and revitalizing his sex drive. Others claimed the contrary, that it could lower his sex drive and thereby relieve all kinds of mental anguish. Until quite recently, most physicians believed that vasectomy could prevent urinary and prostatic disease. Proponents of eugenics saw it as a

*We have made an effort to define the necessary medical terms as they are introduced into the discussion, without becoming encyclopedic. Complete definitions appear in the Glossary.

way to "purify" the genetic composition of the human race. Some advocates of population control have lately portrayed vasectomy as the simplest and easiest method for saving the human race from ecological disaster.

Historical and medical research have shown that these claims were exaggerated, if not downright false, but some of them persist even today. Perhaps the best orientation to vasectomy is a brief tour through the operation's checkered past.

Vasectomy as a Medical Cure

The first human vasectomy was performed in 1894 by a British surgeon in the mistaken belief that it could cure swelling and hardening of the patient's prostate gland. In 1928, an American surgeon performed a vasectomy thinking it would cure impotence. Until very recently, vasectomy was routinely performed on men who were having a diseased prostate gland removed; the idea was to prevent any spreading of prostate infection to the epididymis, the delicate tubule that connects the vas deferens to the testicles (see Figure 2–1 or 2–2). The truth is that except in unusual circumstances vasectomy has no legitimate or necessary medical use other than birth control.

Rejuvenation Through Vasectomy

Other misapplications have gone beyond the province of healing altogether. For centuries, humankind has been searching for eternal life, or a method of prolonging life at least. In 1916, Ludwig Steinach, a brilliant but erratic professor of physiology at the University of Vienna, hypothesized that a man's aging process could be retarded through control of his hormone output. It was known in Steinach's time that the testicles contain two kinds of cells: spermatogenic cells, which produce sperm, and Leydig cells, which produce testosterone, the principal male sex hormone. Testosterone is responsible for a man's secondary sex characteristics: that is, the amount of hair on his body, his sex drive, the pitch of his voice, and the ratio of muscle to fat in his body. Steinach assumed that the amount of testosterone in a man's system controlled the rate at which his body aged and his sexual powers declined. Reasoning that vasectomy would increase a man's output of testosterone, Steinach concluded that it would also promote youthfulness.

He reached that conclusion in the following way: vasectomy traps all of a man's sperm production in his vasa, preventing its release through the penis. Vasectomy must therefore cause some back pressure on the testicles, which in turn discourages the continued production of sperm at high levels and which encourages a diminution of a man's spermatogenic cells. In this assumption he was probably correct. But Steinach further assumed that this diminution of spermatogenic cells would provide room for additional Leydig cells, which would in turn secrete more testosterone, causing a sexual and physical renaissance. Steinach predicted that in a short time after vasectomy, a man would see his hair thicken, his sexual potency increase, and his symptoms of aging or even senility disappear.

Much to the disappointment of those who wish to live forever, Steinach was totally incorrect about the regenerative powers of vasectomy. In his time there was no reliable way to measure hormone output. Today, precise blood-testing techniques show that vasectomy produces no appreciable change in a man's

testosterone level. But the theory caught on. Before
World War II, thousands of men underwent "Steinaching" for the purpose of rejuvenation, and Steinach's
disciples conducted hundreds of studies "proving" that
vasectomized men showed marked improvement in
oxygen intake, muscular firmness, general health, and
startling improvement in sexual potency. Some men
reported an increase in the size of their testicles, others
a decline in symptoms of senility. Rumor has it that
even Steinach's illustrious Viennese neighbor, Sigmund Freud, underwent a Steinaching in hopes of a
longer, more vigorous life. It was not until the 1940s
that Steinach's hypothesis was fully discredited and his
followers were compelled to admit their mistakes.

His legacy of false claims is still with us, if only in a
subtle way. Evan Wylie's widely circulated *Guide to
Voluntary Sterilization* (1973) tells us that "The effect of
vasectomy on a couple's life can be dramatic.... In
one study, three out of four men reported a more active
sex life, although they were at an age when a decline
might have been expected. As to potency, one doctor
who performed some three hundred vasectomies reported that of all his cases, only three reported a loss of
sexual desire or potency after the operation."

And Paul J. Gillette reassures us in his *Vasectomy Information Manual* (1972), saying that "In at least one
large-scale [but uncited] study, a substantial minority
of men reported improved general health after the operation" and that "most couples report after vasectomy
that their sexual rapport has been heightened rather
than diminished." We find it remarkable that vasectomy is still being "marketed" with attractive and misleading promises. In Chapter 5 we will discuss the
sexual improvement that sometimes, but not always,
follows a vasectomy operation. Suffice it to say for now

that vasectomy should be elected for its virtues as a safe and effective form of contraception and for no other reason.

Vasectomy as Social Control

Rejuvenation has not been the most absurd or disturbing misapplication of vasectomy. In 1899, Harry Sharp, M.D., the resident physician at the Jeffersonville Reformatory in Indiana, performed a vasectomy on a young man named Clawson, who had first requested castration. Clawson hoped that castration, the surgical removal of testicles, would help him suppress an uncontrollable impulse to masturbate. Sharp wisely declined to perform the operation but told Clawson a vasectomy would be just as effective in bringing his sex drive under control. When Clawson reported a few months later that he was no longer masturbating, that he was sleeping better, and that his studies had improved, Sharp performed the operation on an additional 175 men who volunteered for it. In 1907, Sharp published a report claiming that "practically every man told me that he sleeps better, feels better, and has a better appetite."

Sharp's patients were obviously as willing as Steinach's to believe that vasectomy had some magical power to affect their sex drive and their health. They stopped or at least reduced their masturbation, even though vasectomy has no significant effect on a man's hormone levels (and therefore no effect on his sex drive). They felt physically healthier because they believed that the operation promoted better health. And if their concentration, schoolwork, and sleep patterns improved, this most likely occurred because the men felt less guilty about their masturbatory behavior. In a

1937 interview, Sharp confessed, "Perhaps I misrepresented the facts ... but we did not know so much about sexual science in those days. I convinced the patient that he would receive all the benefits that could be expected."

Vasectomy and Eugenics

Harry Sharp didn't stop at controlling "excessive" masturbation. In 1909, he reported performing a series of 280 vasectomies for the purpose of eugenic improvement of the human race. Eugenics is the study of human improvement through genetic control: it encourages reproduction among parents with desirable traits and discourages or prohibits reproduction among parents with undesirable traits. Of course, the trick is to decide who defines the term undesirable. Sharp operated on the 280 men because they were found by legal processes to be "defective individuals." Their physical defects included color blindness or poor vision; defects of personality included "selfishness, ingratitude, inconstancy, egotism, and inability to resist any impulse or desire."

Indiana law permitted involuntary sterilization of "defective individuals" to protect the state from having to cope with their offspring. During the 1920s, thirty-one states had similar statutes. In 1927, the United States Supreme Court upheld the eugenic sterilization laws on the grounds that children of the feeble-minded, the insane, and the criminal classes often became wards of the state and thus imposed an unfair burden on normal, law-abiding taxpayers. Justice Oliver Wendell Holmes, speaking for the Court majority, observed that the community has a right, as with compulsory vaccination against smallpox, to inoculate itself against the dependent children of the incompetent and defective.

In the aftermath of World War II and Nazism, a stigma attached to eugenic sterilization, and some legislatures repealed their compulsory sterilization statutes. However, twenty-one states retained these laws, and there have been occasional efforts to renew their enforcement. In 1973, legislators in Tennessee, Mississippi, Ohio, and Illinois introduced bills that would have required compulsory sterilization of welfare parents with two or more children. Vice President Spiro Agnew agreed that government should say, "We're very sorry but we will not be able to allow you to have more children." In California and Oklahoma, judges have agreed to suspend prison terms for men convicted of nonsupport and robbery if they would instead consent to a vasectomy. Nobel laureate in mathematics William Schockley, stepping into the field of eugenics, has advocated paying the mentally retarded a reward if they volunteer for sterilization.

Proposals to sterilize criminals, the retarded, or those who receive public assistance payments have especially outraged leaders of the black community, who have raised questions about the assumptions that underlie the relationship between birth control programs and racial stereotyping. Floyd McKissick, formerly the national director of the Congress of Racial Equality (CORE), has characterized white birth control advocates as having the attitude that "If poor people and Black people just stop having children, the whole problem will go away. In just a few generations, there will be no more poor people and no more Black people —they seem to conceive of birth control as a sort of painless genocide."

McKissick's reference to sterilization as a form of

genocide is a rhetorical overstatement, identifying the birth control movement with Nazi Germany. Experts claim that the Nazis vasectomized as many as one million Europeans for eugenic purposes. Under the provisions of the 1933 Law for the Prevention of Hereditary Disease in Posterity, the German government could order its citizens sterilized for such conditions as schizophrenia, manic depression, or mental retardation. Hereditary diseases such as Huntington's chorea were included on the sterilization list, but so were such conditions as blindness, deafness, and epilepsy, which are rarely inherited. Even persons with harmless deformities such as club foot or dwarfism were subject to sterilization. Nazi Germany was the classic example of a society that went mad trying to "purify" its genetic composition.

Those considered most impure by Nazi ideologists, and thus the most frequent target for sterilization, were the racially "unfit": Jews, Romanian gypsies, and Slavic peoples in general. In addition to vasectomy, Nazi surgeons performed castrations, hysterectomies, and genital mutilations in the name of scientific research. In most cases, the victims were exterminated after the "experiments" were completed. A few survived to tell their story.

Vasectomy and World Population Problems

Since the revelation of these atrocities, national birth control programs have undergone careful scrutiny to insure that they contain no elements of coercion or involuntary recruitment. In 1971, for example, worldwide criticism descended on the government of India for conducting a month-long "vasectomy camp" at Ernakulam in the state of Kerala. As part of a national effort to deal with the crushing problem of overpopulation, the Ernakulam camp vasectomized 63,000 men in its thirty-one days of operation, averaging 2,000 men every twenty-four hours. Ninety-nine surgeons operated day and night, while musical bands and jugglers provided entertainment for those who were waiting their turn. Government-supplied buses shuttled men and their families from outlying villages to the campsite.

Ernakulam's critics were most disturbed by inducements used to get men to "volunteer" for sterilization. The great majority who attended the camp were attracted by the 114-rupee reward (for many, the equivalent of a month's income). The government paid other men to serve as "motivators" and "promoters," offering ten rupees for each "volunteer" they brought to the camp. The motivators apparently compelled men who owed them money to attend the camp and threatened others with physical harm if they did not "volunteer." The motivators brought in old men who were instructed to lie about their age. Several follow-up studies of the psychological effects on men at Ernakulam indicate that a significant minority had never been fully informed of what was going to be done to them. Many claimed they thought they were going to have a simple physical examination. One study revealed that 43 percent of those interviewed later regretted their vasectomies and wished they had not been sterilized (Wolfers and Wolfers, 1974). Equally large percentages reported some decline in health or sex drive, which researchers attribute to the natural decline associated with aging or to the psychological distress of having been involuntarily or semivoluntarily sterilized.

American men whose vasectomies have been truly voluntary report far lower rates of psychological or physical distress, so the effects of vasectomy per se should not be judged on the basis of the Ernakulam studies. However, the episode at Ernakulam highlights the importance of every vasectomy patient giving his voluntary, informed, and rational consent before he undergoes the operation.

Vasectomy as Birth Control: 1960 to the Present

During the 1960s, vasectomy began to emerge in the United States as a popular method of permanent contraception. The Association for Voluntary Sterilization estimated that as late as 1960 only 45,000 American men had undergone voluntary sterilization for contraceptive purposes (although others had undergone vasectomy in conjunction with eugenic sterilization or prostate removal). By the early 1970s, however, approximately three-quarters of a million men per year underwent vasectomy. According to the National Fertility Survey, the number of men electing vasectomy each year leveled off by the mid-1970s to approximately 450,000, where the number remains today. At present, one married couple in eight uses sterilization as their means of birth control.

Several factors account for this sudden growth in vasectomy's popularity during the late 1960s and early 1970s. The women's movement emphasized the need for men and women to share responsibility for contraception. Organizations such as the Association for Voluntary Sterilization, the International Planned Parenthood Federation and Zero Population Growth stepped up their efforts to promote voluntary sterilization as a way to cope with the nation's, and the world's, overpopulation. Hospitals and clinics lowered the barriers against voluntary sterilization, no longer requiring that a man be over the age of thirty-five and have three children before he could obtain a vasectomy. Some hospitals and clinics relaxed rules voluntarily, while others gave in to protests by family planning groups and lawsuits pressed by individuals who had been denied sterilization. During the 1970s a significant number of couples committed themselves to a childless or one-child lifestyle.

The one factor that accounts for most of the increasing number of vasectomies in the early 1970s, however, is the announcement by the United States government in 1969 that the Pill might pose a serious hazard to a woman's health. The government's tests demonstrated that the Pill might cause blood clots and possibly death in an undetermined number of women using it for long periods of time. Many couples between thirty and forty-four years of age, who considered their families complete and were certain they no longer wished to have any (or any additional) children, relied on the Pill —it failed only one user in a hundred—until it was exposed as a significant risk to a woman's health. As we will see in Chapter 7, the only method of contraception that surpasses the Pill in preventing conception is sterilization. The increase in the number of vasectomies and tubal ligations in the early 1970s occurred at the same time that large numbers of couples abandoned the Pill because of its health hazards.

The Lesson of History

At the present time, vasectomy is generally limited to use as an individual means of birth control for men and couples who desire not to have any (more) children. In the years since 1894, almost every other purpose for the operation has been discredited on medical or moral grounds.

2
Male Sexuality, Reproduction, and Vasectomy

Despite vasectomy's current popularity, many individuals are still misinformed about its effect on a man's sexual functioning. The system of glands, organs and tubes that make up the male reproductive tract actually performs three functions: first, enabling a man to produce offspring; second, providing him with a supply of male hormones; and third, enabling him to experience sexual pleasure. Vasectomy affects only the reproductive function; it does not interfere either with his hormone supply or his capacity to give and receive sexual pleasure. A brief sketch of how the three elements of the male sexual system work will make this clear. We will look at the reproductive function first since it is the most immediate concern for anyone contemplating a vasectomy. We will then look at the system's hormonal and sexual functions. Finally, we will describe precisely where and how vasectomy affects or does not affect each of the three functions.

A Functional Map of the System

The glands, organs and tubes that comprise the male reproductive system are located in three parts of the body: the scrotum, the abdomen, and the penis (see Figure 2–1). The scrotum is the sac that holds a man's testicles, each of which serves two functions: producing sperm and producing male hormones. Sperm are the genetic materials of reproduction; hormones are the chemical source of masculine characteristics and the sex drive.

Side View

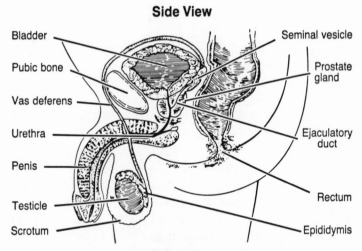

Bladder

Pubic bone

Vas deferens

Urethra

Penis

Testicle

Scrotum

Seminal vesicle

Prostate gland

Ejaculatory duct

Rectum

Epididymis

Figure 2–1
The Male Reproductive Organs

Sperm leave the testicles bathed in testicular fluid, entering the rete testis, a cluster of microscopic tubules at the top of each testicle. From the rete, the sperm move into a tightly coiled, fifteen-foot-long tube called the epididymis. From the epididymis, sperm enter the vas deferens, a fifteen-inch-long tube, about as wide as a venetian blind cord, that rises into the abdomen.

From the vas, sperm and testicular fluid enter the ejaculatory duct, formed by the end of the vas and the exit duct of the seminal vesicle. The seminal vesicle is a gland that produces approximately 65 percent of the fluid called semen. The ejaculatory duct empties into the bulb of the urethra, and it is here that the paths followed by sperm from each testicle first combine. (This area, located near the base of the penis, is sometimes called the bulbous urethra to distinguish it from the part of the urethra that continues as a channel to the tip of the penis.) The mixture of semen is completed by the fluid produced in the prostate gland, which empties into the bulb of the urethra through a separate duct. The process by which sperm, testicular fluid, prostate secretions, and seminal vesicle secretions are moved to and mixed in the bulb is known as emission. During intercourse or masturbation, a man does not become aware of emission through his system until the moment of ejaculatory inevitability, when the fluids are gathered in the bulb. Soon afterward, muscles surrounding the urethra contract rhythmically to cause ejaculation, the sudden spurt of semen that occurs simultaneously with the sensation of sexual pleasure called orgasm.

Sperm Production and Human Reproduction

Testicles

The heart of the male reproductive system is the testicles, which manufacture sperm, the microscopic organisms that carry a man's genetic potential to a woman's unfertilized egg. The testicles of a typical male will produce sperm at a rate of 50,000 per minute —every minute, every day—until he is well into his seventies or beyond. Abraham fathered Isaac at the age of 125; more recently, Charles Chaplin fathered a baby at the age of 80. A man continues to produce millions of sperm each day even after vasectomy, although some experts believe that the rate of sperm production tends to slow somewhat.

Spermatogonia, the primitive cells in the seminiferous tubules from which sperm will eventually form, divide several times before becoming spermatocytes. Spermatocytes undergo further divisions which reduce the chromosome content of sperm to one half that of other body cells. Half of the sperm thus produced contain the genetic coding for a male and half for a female. These immature sperm, called spermatids, do not divide anymore but simply evolve into mature sperm.

Seventy-four days after their birth, sperm leave each testicle via the rete testis. Although sperm leaving the rete testis look mature, they are not yet able to swim on their own nor are they capable of fertilizing a woman's ova or eggs. These abilities will be acquired during the journey through the epididymis (see Figure 2–2).

Epididymis

Each epididymis is a narrow, thin-walled tube fifteen feet in length; it is coiled into a compact mass no larger than a half-inch by two inches and draped over the outside of the testicle. The diameter of the epididymal tubule is 1/200th of an inch, and its walls are only a few cells thick. (The delicacy of the epididymis will be a significant consideration when we examine microsurgical vasectomy reversal in Chapter 8.) The contractions of the epididymis push the maturing sperm along its length in a journey that takes twelve days. The epididymis both secretes and absorbs natural salts and hormones. Although no changes in the appearance of

Front View

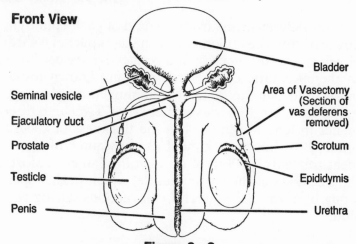

Figure 2–2
The Male Reproductive Organs, Showing Area of Vasectomy

sperm occur during epididymal transit, the special environment of the epididymal fluid either actively promotes or simply allows the sperm to develop the ability to swim and fertilize eggs. In Chapter 8, we will explain why this period of maturation is important for men who remain infertile after a vasectomy reversal attempt.

Vas Deferens

The now-mature sperm enter the vas deferens in preparation for ejaculation. Having developed for three months, they are capable of swimming on their own and fertilizing an egg. Although a man's ejaculate contains hundreds of millions of sperm, they are visible only with the aid of a microscope. Sperm and testicular fluid together contribute only two to five percent to the volume of semen. After vasectomy, when the ejaculate no longer contains these two components, its texture, color, and thickness will appear unchanged.

A vas deferens runs from the end of each epididymis upwards into the abdomen. Each vas is part of a sheath of veins, arteries, nerves, and connective tissues known as the spermatic cord. Some men are known to have more than one vas deferens running through a spermatic cord, but this is extremely rare. Twelve to fifteen inches in length, the vas has the thickness of venetian blind cord, but the channel at the center of the vas measures only 1/100th of an inch in diameter. Most of the thickness of the vas is muscle, which pushes sperm along by means of powerful contractions during emission.

Seminal Vesicles and the Prostate Gland

Each vas deferens empties into an ejaculatory duct. Each duct is formed by the convergence of a vas and the exit duct of a seminal vesicle. Each seminal vesicle secretes a fructose-rich substance that nourishes the sperm and forms the major portion of the ejaculate. The prostate, a gland that surrounds the bladder and produces an additional seminal fluid, has its own exit ducts leading to the bulbous urethra. During emission, most of the fluid in the seminal vesicles and prostate is passed to the urethra in preparation for orgasm. This is why it takes a little while for most men to have a second ejaculation: the seminal vesicles and prostate need time to manufacture and emit more seminal fluids to the urethra. Without the buildup of fluid in the bulb of the urethra, it is difficult to achieve orgasm.

Ejaculation

Contractions of the muscles surrounding the base of the urethra convey semen out of the penis. Technically, ejaculation is the evacuation of semen, while orgasm is the sensation of sexual pleasure that accompanies it. The urethra also conveys urine from the bladder, but in a healthy male, urine and semen will never mix. Since urine can destroy sperm, a powerful sphincter muscle contracts during sexual stimulation, closing down the exit from the bladder to the urethra. This is why it is difficult for a man to urinate when he has an erection.

What Vasectomy Is

Vasectomy is the medical term for the cutting and sealing of the vasa deferentia so that they no longer convey sperm to the ejaculatory ducts. After vasectomy, the seminal vesicles continue to secrete their contents into the ejaculatory ducts and the prostate continues to pass its contents to the urethra. The bulb of the urethra continues to fill with these seminal fluids, causing the pressure that leads to ejaculation, but the ejaculate no longer contains sperm or testicular fluid.

Vasectomy is normally performed in the following manner. A surgeon makes a minor incision on one side of the scrotum and locates the vas deferens. A careful incision into the wall of the cord exposes the vas for clamping at two sites close to each other. The surgeon cuts between the clamps, seals the two ends, and then ties them off for return to the scrotum. The procedure is repeated on the other side of the scrotum.

Vasectomy interrupts the link between the testicles and ejaculatory ducts, but it has no noticeable effect on the overall functioning of the sperm production system. The testicles continue to generate 50,000 sperm per hour. The sperm continue to develop in the seminiferous tubules, and continue to leave the testicles via the

epididymi to enter the vasa. The sperm are blocked at
the site of the vasectomy, where they simply collect
The body's cleansing systems eliminate the sperm by
several methods. The accumulation of sperm in the
vasa creates a back pressure on the epididymi that
may slow production of sperm somewhat. In some
men, the pressure of sperm buildup can reopen a tied
vas, allowing sperm to leak into the scrotum. Sometimes the thinner-walled epididymi give way and develop leaks. In most men, this is not a major concern.
We will have more to say on the subject of postsurgical
medical effects in Chapter 6.

Orgasm

In addition to the production of sperm and hormones,
the male reproductive system serves an erotic function,
providing sexual pleasure through the sensation called
orgasm. Orgasm or climax accompanies ejaculation
and is caused by repeated contractions of the vasa, the
ejaculatory ducts, and the urethra. Vasectomy has no
effect on orgasm.

Sexual Stimulation and Orgasm

Sexual excitement in a man, caused by physical or
mental stimulation, is manifested when his penis
becomes erect. Delicate sphincter valves that normally
close off the tiny blood vessels in the muscles of the
penis suddenly open, allowing an infusion of blood that
distends the penis and makes it erect. Physical stimulation of the penis triggers the release of a substance
called norepinephrine, which sets off contractions in
the vasa, ejaculatory ducts, seminal vesicles, and prostate gland, which in turn cause emission of the seminal
fluids, sperm, and testicular fluid to the bulb of the

urethra. Orgasm occurs when the muscles that surround the urethra finally expel the semen.

Orgasm After Vasectomy

Since the testicles and vasa supply only sperm and testicular fluid to the ejaculate—a mere two to five percent of the total volume—vasectomy does not alter a man's sensation of orgasm. The absence of sperm and testicular fluid does not alter the color, texture, or thickness of the ejaculate in any discernible way. As we shall see in Chapter 5, any decrease in sexual pleasure after vasectomy is almost always the result of some difficulty in adapting psychologically to sterility rather than physiological change.

Male Hormones

The third function of the male reproductive system is manufacture of male hormones (androgens), which at puberty trigger the growth of a male's pubic hair and the sprouting of his beard. It accounts as well for the change in his voice, the bulking and strengthening of his muscles, and the awakening of his sex drive. Once he has matured, a continuous flow of testosterone and other androgens from his testicles helps maintain the metabolic balance characteristic of males.

Castration, removal of the testicles, renders a man a eunuch. Once his body no longer has a source of androgens, a male will lose his facial hair, will often lose his ability to have an erection, and will find that his voice sounds more feminine. In the Middle Ages, young boys were castrated so that they could sing the soprano parts in church choirs, and sheiks castrated harem guards so that they would not present competition for the women's sexual favors. Since vasectomy interferes with the male reproductive function, it has sometimes been confused with castration.

Vasectomy has none of the hormonal effects of castration. With or without vasectomy, the testicles distribute testosterone to the body through the bloodstream, not through the vas deferens, which transports only sperm. Vasectomy neither increases nor diminishes the testicles' ability to produce and distribute male hormones. Vasectomy may have other effects on the body, particularly the immune system, but we will look more closely at the possibility of this side effect in Chapter 6.

Vasectomy as Permanent Contraception

Of our several goals in this brief introduction, the first has been to assure you that vasectomy has no noticeable impact on a man's ability to perform sexually or, barring psychological difficulties, on his ability to enjoy sex fully. It will not affect the balance of male hormones, masculine characteristics, or sex drive. Nor should it make him feel any different physically from the way he felt before his operation.

It will, however, make him sterile—unable to procreate through intercourse. This is not to say that he cannot be a father, by adopting a child or becoming a step-parent. But we want to emphasize the permanence of this sterility, especially now that we are ready to discuss the process that a man or couple should follow in deciding whether vasectomy is the appropriate form of birth control. In practical terms, vasectomy must be considered permanent because reversal is so difficult. Recall that the inner channel of the vas deferens is only 1/100th of an inch in diameter: the inner and outer diameters must be joined such that there is absolutely no leaking from the point of reconnection.

In Chapter 8, we will examine some of the impressive —let us say miraculous—advances in microsurgery that have made it possible for more than half of the men who wish to reverse vasectomy to become fertile again. However, reversal is still far from perfect. We therefore urge every man or couple contemplating a vasectomy to consider it an irrevocable step. While vasectomy will probably not alter a man's sex life and certainly will not change the hormonal balance in his body, it will end his fertility forever unless good fortune and a skillful microsurgeon make it possible for him to regain it. We recommend that you make your decision on vasectomy a careful one, a decision you can live with for the rest of your life.

3
Is Vasectomy Right for You?

Although you or your partner may now be considering vasectomy for contraception, you need to figure out whether it is the right choice for you in the current context of your life. You may already have sought advice about vasectomy from your doctor, a counselor, a friend, or a member of your family. You are no doubt aware that everyone has biases and preferences when it comes to fertility, contraception, and childbearing. This makes your problem of deciding whom to take advice from even more difficult.

Before offering you any personal advice, we would like to make our own position clear. We believe that vasectomy is a safe and effective form of birth control, but it is not appropriate for everyone. It is a reasonable choice for those individuals whose circumstances make them ready for permanent birth control—the emphasis being on the word *permanent*. If you choose either vasectomy or tubal ligation as your form of contraception, you are saying in effect that your place in the life cycle, your commitment to your current relationship, or the needs and wishes of your family make it highly unlikely that you will want any (more) children.

If you are single and childless and plan to remain that way, the decision to have yourself sterilized is entirely your own. However, the great majority of men who seek vasectomy are married and have been for ten years or more, or have been in a stable relationship. Usually it is a decision that a couple must reach together, and in doing so they must answer two questions: is it time for us to be using permanent birth control? and, if it is, which of us should be sterilized? Given the symbolic importance placed on fertility and sexuality in our society, not to mention the dynamics of your relationship or your feelings about yourself, it is little wonder that the relatively simple surgical procedures of interrupting a man's vasa deferentia or a woman's fallopian tubes can become so emotionally charged.

Children play important symbolic roles in a parent's life. They represent our link to the future, our only means to immortality on earth. They are the visible proof of the bond between a man and a woman. For some men, they are the ultimate proof of virility. Above all, children give parents a unique opportunity to love and be loved in return. Thus a man or a couple's decision not to have any or any more children is filled with meaning for both partners, as well as for any children they might already have.

For a man, vasectomy should be a strong statement about his commitment to the future. He should be saying that he, his partner, and any new partner he might have in the future will not have a child from that time forward. When the decision to have a vasectomy is made in the context of a full family discussion, sterilization can draw a family closer together, ratifying their sense of unity and completeness. It can be a way for a father to say that he wants to devote his time, income, and energy to the children he has, or to himself and his mate.

Two British experts on the psychology of vasectomy (Wolfers and Wolfers, 1974) have said, "There is one and only one reason for a man to undergo this operation, and that is that for his own sake, and for mature and informed reasons, he no longer wishes to have any (more) children." We agree with this statement, as far as it goes. Vasectomy decisions always affect a couple and a family. Such a decision crystallizes their past, their present, and their future. In a family system, there are very few things that an individual can do "for his own sake," that do not have some impact on the lives of others. This chapter—and this book—are not written strictly for the sovereign male.

At this point, you may be a bit disoriented by our approach. We have implied that you will be making a decision about the appropriateness of vasectomy to your circumstances without first telling you how safe the operation is, how it compares to other methods of birth control, or exactly how it can be reversed. We will instead be asking you to consider the stability of your marriage and your relationship to your children (if you have any). In a real sense, these are the most important elements in your decision. The information about the safety or effectiveness of vasectomy is more or less technical, and it becomes important only after you have decided you are ready to use permanent birth control. Information on the medical and psychological aftereffects of vasectomy can be found in Chapters 5 and 6, and a comparison of vasectomy to other means of birth control can be found in Chapter 7, but the information about your attitudes toward your relationship and toward the future can only be found inside yourself.

Even the most stable and contented couples, fully committed to their future together, assume some risks when they adopt sterilization as their means of birth control. None of us can predict the future. When a couple contemplates a vasectomy or a tubal ligation, they must force themselves to imagine things that they doubtless prefer not to think about: how each would feel if the other died or if they got divorced; whether, if they remarried, they would want a child with their new spouse; and whether they would want another child if one or all of their children died. At the same time, few of us can afford to live out our lives waiting for the worst to happen. We prepare for the future by assuming that tomorrow will be pretty much like today. We only have to be aware of that assumption.

While you cannot predict or control the future, you can take responsibility for your choices. You can begin by asking questions. What are the reasons for believing that you are finished wanting children, and why are you unlikely to change your mind even if circumstances change? You can make an assessment of the current state of your marriage or relationship and of its likelihood to survive over the next ten or twenty years. You can look inside yourself to discover how you feel about your body and the meaning of your fertility.

To assist you in making these judgments, we have designed a self-evaluation that appears in the next section. Worked out with the advice of psychologists and family counselors, it will help you get in touch with your attitudes and with those of your partner. We think it is a good way to approach the process of mutual decision making. When you have completed the self-evaluation, we will suggest some further steps to take before settling on your decision.

Vasectomy Readiness Self-Evaluation: Introduction

This self-evaluation is not a conventional test. There is no score on this test that will tell you whether or not you are ready for a vasectomy. The questions have been designed to start discussion between you and your partner. Later they will help you focus on the important issues when you broaden your consultation to a circle that includes your physician, and, if appropriate, a family counselor.

How to Take This Test

We propose that you set aside a quiet time to complete the self-evaluation: perhaps as much as two hours, when you are unlikely to be interrupted or distracted. If you are reading this book with your partner, you may want to make a copy of the questionnaire so that each of you can work on it separately. But work on it at the same time, so you can get together while the answers are still fresh in both your minds. You may want to exchange your written answers, or you may simply choose to discuss your feelings and reactions.

If you are anything like us, you would probably prefer not to go through the trouble of writing out your answers. Nevertheless we urge you to write out your answers. You can talk or think out your answers, but writing them out insures that your reasoning is solid rather than sketchy. Written answers can be reviewed later, when you are in a different mood.

When you feel the time is right, grab this book, a pen or pencil, and some sheets of lined paper; take the phone off the hook, sit down at a table, and focus on your inner self.

A Special Word to Childless Couples and Single Men

The questions in the self-evaluation have been formulated as if respondents were married (or in a stable relationship) with one or more children. The questions are relevant for couples who have not yet had children, and many are relevant for single men who think they might marry, even if this currently seems a remote possibility. We suggest that you complete the self-evaluation if you are contemplating a vasectomy as a birth control option, regardless of your marital or parental status. In the concluding sections of this chapter, we will discuss some of the important decision-making factors that affect childless couples and single men.

Interpreting Your Answers

There is no right or wrong to the questions you have just grappled with. Moreover, it is not possible for us to explore every reason why a couple might seek vasectomy as their means of birth control or to anticipate every concern a man might have before deciding on vasectomy. We can only offer a framework within which you can locate your reasons for considering it. However, we believe this framework can be very useful to you in assessing the appropriateness of vasectomy to your circumstances.

The Range of Responses

Our personal and clinical experiences, interviews with vasectomized men, and analysis of psychological

THE VASECTOMY
READINESS SELF-EVALUATION

Is Vasectomy Right for You?

A. Your Current Contraceptive(s)

1. At present, who is responsible for birth control in your relationship, you or your partner? What method(s) are you using?

2. Do you consider the method(s) effective; foolproof?

3. Do you consider the method(s) safe from a health perspective?

4. Have the two of you experienced any pregnancies while using your current method(s) of birth control?

5. Does your current means of contraception interfere with sexual pleasure?

6. Have you been raised to believe that mechanical or surgical forms of birth control are unnatural or sinful? If so, do you still believe this is true?

B. Your Health/Your Body

7. How would you rate your personal health at this moment: excellent, good, fair, or poor? Do you suffer from any serious or chronic diseases? How is your partner's overall health: excellent, good, fair, or poor? Does your partner suffer from any serious disease?

   For men: a. What impact do you think a vasectomy is likely to have on your personal health: positive, negative, no change? On your emotional well-being: positive, negative, no change?

b. Does your partner suffer from any physical or mental condition that would make a pregnancy hazardous to her health? Her well-being?

For women: **a.** What impact do you think a vasectomy would have on your partner's physical health: positive, negative, no change? On his emotional well-being: positive, negative, no change?

b. What impact do you think a pregnancy would have on your physical health? On your emotional well-being?

C. Timing

8. Who first suggested that you consider vasectomy as your method of contraception?

9. What important events were happening in your personal or family life at the time the topic of vasectomy first arose? Had you switched contraceptives for other than medical reasons? Had you gone through pregnancy, childbirth, or abortion? Had you or any member of your family been through a period of financial stress? Were you having marital conflicts? If so, did they have anything to do with sex?

D. Your Relationship

10. How would you rate your current marriage or relationship: excellent, good, indifferent, troubled?

11. How would you rate your sexual satisfaction within your relationship or marriage: excellent, good, indifferent, troubled?

12. In the past year, have you suffered from any sexual performance problems (for men, impotence or premature ejaculation; for women, inability to reach orgasm)? Have you lost any of your interest in sexual relations? Has your partner lost interest in sexual relations? If yes to either one, why do you think this is so?

For men: a. If you were to have a vasectomy, do you think you would enjoy sex with your wife or partner more, less, or the same?

b. Do you think she would enjoy having sex with you more if you had a vasectomy? Do you believe a fear of pregnancy seriously inhibits her desire to have sex with you?

For women: a. If your partner were to have a vasectomy, do you think you would enjoy sex with him more, less, or the same? Do you think it would make him more attractive to you?

b. If he had a vasectomy, do you think it would make him enjoy having sex with you more, or would it make no difference?

13. Have extramarital affairs or outside relationships been an issue?

For men: a. If you were to have a vasectomy, do you think other women will find you more attractive, less attractive, or unchanged? Do you think your partner considers this an important issue?

b. If you have a vasectomy, are you more likely to have an affair with another woman, or will it make no difference?

For women: a. If your partner has a vasectomy, do you think other women will find him more attractive or less attractive, or will it make no difference?

b. If he has a vasectomy, will it make him more likely or less likely to have an affair with another woman, or will it make no difference?

E. Thinking About Your Family and Future

14. Do you consider your current family complete? Do you now have all the children you will ever want? Does your partner consider the family complete, and does he or she have all the children he or she will ever want?

15. If you were to divorce in the next five years, do you think you would remarry? If you did, would you be likely to want to have a child with your new partner?

16. If you were to divorce in the next five years, do you think your partner might remarry and want to have a child with his or her new partner?

17. If you were to die in the next five years, might your partner want to remarry and have a child? If your partner were to die, might you want to remarry and have a child?

18. If one or all of your children were to die, do you think that you would want to have another child?

studies persuades us that there is an ideal reason for seeking a vasectomy: that a *couple* sees the operation in a positive sense as a mutual commitment to their already successful marriage or relationship. Such a couple considers their family complete, whether it comprises just the two of them or just the two of them plus eight children. Their decision to switch over to permanent birth control is a way of saying they are dedicated to maintaining their family as it exists today.

Our notion of the ideal may be controversial in some circles. Unlike some advocates, we do not consider nuisance value: annoyance with a mechanical means of contraception such as a condom, diaphragm, or foam is not by itself a sufficient reason to terminate fertility. Nor do we have much tolerance for the approach that asks whose "turn" it is to take responsibility for contraception. In practical terms, male contraception is limited to coitus interruptus (withdrawal before orgasm), condoms, and vasectomy; neither of the first two is completely efficient at preventing pregnancy. If it becomes the man's "turn" to practice contraception, he is consigned to a vasectomy by default. We believe contraception is a mutual responsibility that one party in a relationship carries out for the benefit of both. Thus vasectomy should be adopted only when both parties agree fully that they no longer want to have children.

The Negative Extreme

If commitment to a marriage or relationship represents the best possible reason to seek vasectomy, the use of sterilization as a weapon in marital or sexual conflict represents the worst. This is true for vasectomy or tubal ligation. As we have already noted, vasectomy is sometimes associated with powerful social and psychological meanings—castration, power-lessness, loss of masculinity—and thus it can become a devastating weapon. We know of a wife who pressured her husband to have a vasectomy soon after she learned of his having an affair; as the husband later confessed, he consented to the operation in the hope that she would interpret it as an act of penance. Another man told us he had a vasectomy to silence his wife, who had been through the rigors of an unwanted pregnancy and childbirth. A third individual told us that he under-went vasectomy because he felt that the birth of an-other child would completely entrap him in a marriage that he had not yet mustered the courage to leave.

None of these motives constitutes a valid ground for relinquishing fertility, or for insisting that your spouse do so. A gesture of self-sacrifice will not hold a failing relationship together. And you might want to have chil-dren with a future partner. Vasectomy or tubal ligation should be understood as a means to prevent pregnancy, never as a cure for a failing relationship. If you sus-pect after taking the self-evaluation that your interest in vasectomy may involve a weakness rather than strength in your relationship, we urge you to seek family counseling first. The final section of this chapter will cover family counseling; for now, let us take a clos-er look at each of the five sections of the self-evaluation.

Section A: Your Current Contraceptive(s)

If you were using your current method of birth con-trol with complete confidence and enjoyment, you probably wouldn't be reading this. Dissatisfaction might stem from your fear that your contraceptive will fail, that it might pose a threat to your health or the health of the person you love, or that it is too much of a bother to use on a regular basis. In general, we suggest that you consider all the effective, safe, and fairly convenient methods of contraception surveyed in Chapter 7 before deciding on permanent birth control.

Is a previous failure of your contraceptive valid grounds for ending your fertility? An unplanned pregnancy can represent a serious emotional and financial setback for a couple who no longer want children. For many, deciding whether to go through with the pregnancy or seek an abortion represents a crisis of values; it is important to them that they never be forced to make that choice. As many as 40 percent of couples seeking vasectomy may have experienced a failure with a nonpermanent means of contraception (Ager, et al., 1974).

Couples who have experienced contraceptive failure should ask themselves whether they were using one of the maximally effective, nonpermanent forms of contraception when the pregnancy occurred. If you were relying on a condom or a diaphragm, you might want to try the Pill or an IUD. (For women over thirty-five, or smokers, the Pill probably represents too great a medical risk.) If contraceptive failure occurred while you were using an IUD or the Pill, and you are convinced that you want no more pregnancies, you are probably a very good candidate for surgical birth control.

Some people contemplate vasectomy when use of a condom, diaphragm, or foam interferes with their enjoyment of sex. As we hinted earlier, we are uncomfortable with the idea that a couple would foreclose on their future for the sake of sexual convenience. The Pill or an IUD allows the same spontaneity during foreplay as sterilization. While neither the Pill nor an IUD is quite as effective or safe as vasectomy, they are not permanent. Freedom from distraction during lovemaking is a nice but decidedly secondary benefit of vasectomy; it should not be your primary motive for the operation.

Section B: Your Health/Your Body

We asked you to look at your sense of your body and your overall health, and do the same for your partner, for two reasons. Research indicates that a man who feels significant concern about his physical health or the integrity of his body is likely to have a difficult time adjusting psychologically to vasectomy. This seems also to be true of men with highly developed fears for their partner's health. If you recognize either of these characteristics in yourself, please consult a counselor before seeking a vasectomy.

Our questions are also meant to help you determine whether you are contemplating vasectomy as a way to make a sacrifice for your partner's health or emotional stability. Certainly there are women for whom pregnancy, childbirth, and childrearing pose serious, even life-threatening hazards, but the number is actually quite small. If pregnancy would threaten a woman's health, she should be the one to consider sterilization first unless her gynecologist or psychiatrist recommends otherwise. If a man undergoes vasectomy, not because he is convinced that he is finished wanting children but because he wants to protect his wife or lover, he runs the risk of feeling that she can never fully appreciate his sacrifice. Gratitude can be deadly. We will have more to say on the issue of who is the better candidate for sterilization in Chapter 7.

Section C: Timing

Since vasectomy is permanent, it should not be thought of as a way to cope with short-term problems.

If you are passing through a period of curable illness or temporary financial crisis, if a member of your family has died, or if you have just had a child, you might reasonably wait a year to see whether you still feel that your decision would be permanent. Gynecologists recommend waiting a year after childbirth for tubal ligation, long enough to make sure the newborn is normal and healthy. These guidelines apply just as well to recent fathers who are considering vasectomy. We would also suggest a year's wait for individuals or couples in marriage counseling or psychotherapy, since there is a great likelihood that this experience will lead to major reevaluations of current circumstances and future options.

D: Your Relationship

We have offered it as general guidance that a decision on vasectomy should be reached in light of the long-term prospects of a relationship. Here we narrow the focus to two crucial issues: sexual relations and trust.

In the area of sexual relations, we can tell you that vasectomy is not a cure for sexual performance problems in a man or a cure for frigidity in a woman. Concern about the possibility of pregnancy can interfere with the spontaneity of sex, making a couple reluctant to indulge in sexual relations around the time the female is ovulating. Studies on the subject indicate that for couples who already enjoy each other sexually, the sense of freedom after vasectomy may well enhance their pleasure (Ferber, et al., 1967; Leavesley, 1980). But if a woman has lost interest totally in having intercourse with her husband or lover, the cause almost invariably runs deeper than fear of a pregnancy.

The same is true when a man suffers from impotence or premature ejaculation. As a first step, he should see a urologist to determine whether the source of his impotence is organic: a urologist will order endocrine tests to measure whether the male's testosterone levels are too low to sustain his sex drive. In a majority of cases, however, impotence is caused by anxiety, alienation, or suppressed anger. It is often the signal that a relationship is under great stress. Vasectomy is not a good idea while a couple is struggling with any sort of anguish, but impotence and vasectomy are an especially bad mix because of the operation's symbolic association with castration and weakness.

Then there is trust. We live in a time of rapidly changing values, particularly about marriage and relationships, and many couples seem not to expect the strict adherence to monogamy that was the rule for earlier generations. In addition, there are more single adults in our society than ever before, and many value the freedom to experience a number of sexual relationships. In keeping with these trends, various organizations promoted vasectomy in the 1960s on the grounds that it would make a man more attractive to women who were looking for a one-night stand. Among couples, married or living together, who expect that they will remain sexually faithful to each other, some women fear that vasectomy may make their partner more attractive to other women and encourage outside affairs. Some men, in fact, have told researchers that they elected vasectomy because they anticipated becoming promiscuous.

Research completed in the mid-1970s (Maschhoff, et al., 1976) indicates that married men who have been sterilized are no more likely to indulge in extramarital sex than their fertile counterparts. Whether this remains true today is open to question. Our guess is that things have not changed that much.

What counts is not statistics but your feelings about yourself and your partner. Do you have a reliable basis for trust? The two of you can discuss your fears, hopes, and expectations in this area on your own; we just wanted to make certain you put it on your agenda.

Section E: Thinking About Your Family and Future

Throughout this chapter, we have been asking you to determine, in your present state of mind, whether you are finished having pregnancies. Minimally, we have asked you to think about whether you are finished having children together, assuming you are married or in a stable relationship. Here we ask you to think about how you would feel if the future was unlike the present, how you would feel if life forced you through a painful change. No one marries expecting to divorce. No one likes to imagine a lover's death or how it would feel having children with another partner. Above all, no father or mother can really bear the thought of a child—or all of their children—dying. Yet nightmares sometimes come true—bad things happen to good people every day.

There is no sure way to know how you would feel about sterility if you were to get divorced, if your loved ones were to die, or if you were to fall in love with another person one, five, or ten years from now. You could try to adopt a child. You could try artificial insemination (in Chapter 10, we discuss its limitations). Probably the best way to know if you would regret a vasectomy is to ask yourself the question and listen to what your feelings tell you.

A Question for the Childless Couple

Up to our discussion of Section E, everything we have said so far applies to couples without children as well as those who have children. There are actually two kinds of "childless" couples: those who have never had children and those who have children from previous relationships (i.e., they have had no children by each other). For the latter group, vasectomy seems to be a popular choice when both parties are past thirty-five and neither is interested in adding to their new family.

The issues are more difficult when a young couple, married for the first and (they assume) only time, chooses sterilization as their form of contraception. This couple must make a special effort to understand the mutual commitment vasectomy calls for, more so than a couple who already have children. To see this point, you might imagine the case of a man with children who has a vasectomy sometime before his wife divorces him. If he remarries, and a vasectomy reversal fails, he is still a parent and always will be. Now imagine that man in the same circumstance, except that he never was a father. His wife can become a parent with a new husband or lover; unless he is fortunate and can have his vasectomy reversed, he can never choose to become a natural parent. Certainly, we do not mean that both partners in a childless marriage should have themselves sterilized so that one will have no advantage over the other after a divorce. This example is meant to illuminate the meaning of the word *permanent*.

Vasectomy and the Single Man

Two types of single men might consider vasectomy. With the first type, a man formerly married and the father of one or more children, the issues are straight-forward: do you consider yourself finished having children regardless of whether or not you remarry? If you have just gotten out of a marriage or long-standing relationship, we would urge you to wait at least a year before going ahead with a vasectomy. Your view of male/female relationships may change as the bitterness or anguish of separation fades.

For the younger man, particularly one who has never been married, the questions to be asked reach to the unknowable: how will he feel when he is forty or fifty years old about never having been a parent? What if he meets a woman in only ten years whom he loves so much that he wants to have a child with her?

Physicians are generally reluctant to tell a patient what he should or shouldn't do in matters not directly pertaining to his physical survival in the presence of disease. However, many follow their conscience and refuse to perform vasectomies on men in their twenties who have never been fathers. They are also reluctant when the reason for requesting sterilization is to help in solving the world's population problem. Vasectomy should be a personal, not a political statement. Most physicians believe that it should in most cases be performed only toward the second half of the life cycle, when a man has given life to all the children he will ever want—something that can only be known by experience. In sum, they are rightly cautious with young men who believe their feelings won't change in twenty years.

On the other hand, a single, childless male over the age of twenty-one need not despair of finding a urologist who will perform a vasectomy. We believe that if you are thoughtfully committed to having the operation, you are entitled to a vasectomy. Most family planning clinics will honor your request under the same condition. Some men have made a convincing argument that the certainty of surgical contraception makes it possible for them to contemplate marriage and a stable family life, a step they would not otherwise take because of their desire not to have children. Others have pointed out that they simply have a right to determine how they will live out their own future.

Taking the Next Step

Now that you have evaluated your readiness for vasectomy, you have probably decided one of three things: that vasectomy is not for you; that you would like to talk to a marriage counselor before you seek the services of a surgeon; or that you are certain vasectomy makes sense for you. If you fall into the first category, you might turn to Chapters 7 and 10 for advice on contraceptive alternatives to vasectomy. If you fall into the second category, you can check the List of Counseling Services at the back of the book to locate a qualified counselor or therapist. And if you fall into the last category, your next step is probably to the telephone to make an appointment with a urologist or family planning clinic. But read on.

A Word of Advice About Advice

Many couples receive prevasectomy counseling only from their urologist. Urologists have a great deal of experience and knowledge of vasectomy, but they are usually not trained to recognize marital issues or stresses that lurk behind a request for vasectomy. Nor do they have unlimited time for counseling sessions before you decide whether or not you want the operation.

While urologists deserve respect as medical professionals, they will be the first to concede they are not psychologists or social workers.

We have urged you to seek professional advice if you experienced any confusion or disagreement with your partner while completing the self-evaluation. If you feel reasonably certain at this point that vasectomy would be right for you, we still recommend that you consult a marriage or family counselor. We need to distinguish here between marriage or family counselors on the one hand and family planning counselors on the other.

Family planning counselors usually work out of birth control clinics. While they are professionals, their expertise centers on contraceptive choices rather than the broad-based, general-counseling topics of concern to all members of a family—including your children. A decision about vasectomy is really a decision about the present and future of your entire family, not simply which method of birth control is most efficient or safe. The counseling you are likely to receive at a family planning clinic is not as extensive or thorough as the exploration that a marriage or family counselor can help you undertake.

We have another reservation about the counseling atmosphere at family planning clinics. They function in a dual capacity. On the one hand, their mission is to provide gynecological, urological, and contraceptive services to individuals and couples. On the other, they are committed to contributing to the solution of the world's population problem. These goals may be in conflict, particularly if a couple is ambivalent about permanent contraception. Counselors must beware of pushing sterilization as a way to promote the clinic's higher purposes—possibly helping the world a little at great cost to the individual.

We worry about promotion generally when the issue is sterilization. The *Boston Globe* sports section recently carried an ad for a well-known chain of family planning clinics that asked, "Are You Man Enough to Have a Vasectomy?" We seriously doubt that a man should be asked to settle the issue of his fertility because of a dare in the sports section. The bottom line for a family planning clinic should reflect stable, happy families.

Whether you obtain your vasectomy from a clinic or private urologist is your choice. The next chapter includes advice on how to choose between them. We recommend that your decision-making process include a marriage or family counselor.

4
The Vasectomy Experience

This chapter is addressed to the potential vasectomy candidate. It will help you decide whether to employ the services of a private urologist or a family planning clinic. It will help you anticipate the operation physically and mentally, including the before and after procedures. It contains important information on the steps to take until you are assured that you are no longer fertile, in case you prove to be one of the rare individuals who experiences vasectomy failure.

The Operation Itself

A vasectomy is a relatively simple procedure that normally takes less than thirty minutes. First, you will be asked to exchange your clothes for the characteristically skimpy hospital gown and lie on a surgical table. In a urologist's office, you may be asked to undress only from the waist down. If you have not already done so before your arrival, your doctor or his or her assistant will shave your scrotum and paint it with an antiseptic solution such as iodine, hexachlorophene, or alcohol. The surgeon begins by gently exploring one side of the scrotum above your testicle. This procedure locates your vas deferens and determines the exact spot for the incision. With a very fine needle the surgeon injects a local anesthetic into the skin overlying the vas and into the deeper tissue surrounding it. The local anesthetic takes effect in less than a minute. All vasectomy incisions are made fairly high up on the scrotum, because at this location the vasa are close to the surface and because this procedure avoids the possibility of damaging the testicles or epididymis.

After the incision, your surgeon will inject more local anesthetic into the tissue around the vas deferens and into its sheath. You may feel a slight burning sensation and perhaps a dull ache. Once the vas deferens has been identified, the surgeon stabilizes it with a clamp and makes a vertical cut into its sheath, taking care to avoid any of the large blood vessels or nerves near the vas. Any small vessels that bleed are sealed off by electrocauterizing them or by tying them with a fine thread. Sealing off these loose blood vessels helps prevent the postoperative complication of hematoma, a painful accumulation of blood in the scrotum.

Once the sheath has been opened, and the vas deferens exposed, the surgeon pulls a short loop of the vas out of its sheath. Drawing out the vas will likely cause some dull aching in your groin or lower abdomen and may give you a feeling of queasiness or nausea. This sensation usually lasts only a moment or so. The surgeon cuts through the vas, leaving it in two sections. Some surgeons prefer simply to cut through the vas, removing none of its length. Others will remove a quarter- to half-inch segment of vas and send it to a lab for positive identification, making certain that the vas and not a blood vessel or nerve cord has been cut. Other physicians, although fewer than was once true, remove segments of vas anywhere from one to six inches in length.

How much, if any, of the vas is removed has important implications for the future. The cut ends of the vas can spontaneously reconnect themselves in a process called recanalization, which is more likely to occur when no additional segment has been removed. As you might expect, removing none of the vas also allows the best chance of surgical reconnection if you decide to have your vasectomy reversed. However, you will want to be aware that removal of a quarter- to half-inch of vas lowers the chance of recanalization, has little effect on your chances for surgical reconnection, and does allow for positive identification in a laboratory. Removing very long segments lowers the probability of recanalization to near-zero, but also destroys the possibility of surgical reconnection, in addition to increasing the likelihood of postoperative complications. We strongly recommend that you have only a small segment of vas removed for positive identification.

Sealing the ends of the vasa is another topic you may wish to discuss in advance with your surgeon. A few physicians do not secure the ends of the vasa in any way so as to promote the best chance of success in a reversal operation. However, this procedure significantly increases the chance of spontaneous recanalization, even when long segments of the vasa have been removed. In addition, it always results in the formation of granulomas, or sperm-filled cysts, at the vasectomy site. Granulomas, occasionally painful, may require later surgical removal.

The most common method for securing the ends of the vas is tying them off, or ligating them. However, simply tying the ends seems to produce a slightly higher recanalization rate than other sealing methods, such as clips or fulguration (the electrocauterization of the ends). Sealing the ends of the vas with clips is an easy, effective method with a low recanalization rate, but it seems to do some damage to vas tissue, lowering the chances of reversal.

Fulguration involves the insertion of an electrocautery needle into the inner diameter of each of the cut ends of the vasa. Burning the inner lining of the vas produces scarring, which shuts down the open ends. After both ends have been fulgurated, only one of them is placed back in the spermatic cord sheath, and the sheath is then sealed with a metal clip or suture. With this method of sealing and separating the two ends of the vas, the chances of recanalization appear to be near zero, and a minimum of tissue damage results. Fulguration seems to strike the balance between preventing recanalization and preserving your chances for subsequent reversal.

Once the ends of the vas have been sealed, your surgeon will search carefully for any bleeding vessels, staunching them with electrocautery or surgical thread. He or she then places the ends of the vas back in the scrotum and closes the incision with self-absorbing sutures that dissolve on their own in a week, with non-absorbable sutures that will be removed in five to seven days, or with no sutures. We prefer a surgical method that employs only quarter-inch incisions in the scrotum and no sutures. These small wounds usually seal themselves in less than a day, becoming virtually invisible within two weeks. Since these incisions remain open, blood and serum are less likely to accumulate and a hematoma is less likely to result. After your surgeon is finished operating on both sides of your scrotum, he or she will apply sterile gauze to your wounds.

Choosing Between a Private Doctor and a Clinic

Although vasectomy is a relatively simple procedure, you will want to feel certain that you are in the care of a skilled, experienced surgeon, one who understands the surgical and emotional dimensions of the operation. Generally speaking, you have two choices: a private urologist or a family planning clinic, some of which are private, some nonprofit, and some associated with a hospital's department of reproductive medicine. Clinics almost always have a staff of family planning counselors in addition to urologists (physicians who specialize in surgery on the male reproductive tract). Occasionally, family practitioners or general surgeons will have experience doing vasectomies, but more than likely they will refer you to a private urologist or to a clinic.

You can decide for yourself which you prefer. The cost of vasectomy at a clinic is usually between $150 and $200, while private urologists usually charge between $250 and $300. In some states, all or part of these costs may be covered by medical insurance.

At a clinic, you may not meet your surgeon until the day of your operation. You will interview with one of the staff counselors, who are trained to provide you with general information about the procedural aspects and effectiveness of vasectomy. The counselors are also responsible for screening out applicants who show signs of emotional or marital problems. In some clinics, your initial interview will be conducted in a group. Clinics usually have well-equipped operating

rooms, similar to those in a hospital outpatient department; of course, clinics located in hospitals are likely to
be very well equipped.

Private urologists work out of their office or a hospital outpatient department rather than as employees of
a clinic. While their fees are somewhat higher than
those at a clinic, they are likely to spend more time
with a man or a couple, trying to assess whether vasectomy is the right form of birth control for them.

The Initial Interview

Whether you choose a private physician or a clinic, a
vasectomy will not be performed during your initial
visit. Almost every urologist or clinic uses this visit for
interviewing and for giving information about the operation to the candidate and his partner. The candidate
will be asked to go home for at least a week to think
over his decision; the urologist or counselor uses this
time to reflect on his or her assessment of the candidate. New York State recently passed a law requiring a
vasectomy candidate to wait a month between his initial interview and surgery. If your doctor or counselor
has doubts about the appropriateness of the operation
in your circumstances, you may be asked to consult a
psychiatrist or marriage counselor before surgery is
performed, or you may be asked to wait a year before
returning for another evaluation.

The interview begins with the urologist or counselor
gathering information from you about your general
health. If you are married or in a stable relationship,
your partner will likely be asked to attend this interview also. You will be asked whether you would feel
the same way about not having children if the two of
you were parted by divorce or death, or if any children
you now have were to die. You have already learned a

great deal about your feelings from the self-evaluation in the previous chapter, so there should be few surprises at your interview.

During your initial interview, you will have the opportunity to get answers to some of the important questions you may have about the operation. If you have chosen a private urologist, you can discuss with your doctor how the operation is to be performed. While you are there to convince the urologist or counselor that you are a clear-thinking candidate for sterilization, you are also a consumer of medical services with a right to know exactly what is going to happen to you before, during, and after your surgery.

This opportunity in the initial interview to discuss the options with your physician, well in advance of the surgery, is the main advantage of going to a private urologist. You can talk over your concerns and preferences as to surgical technique: how much of the vasa should be removed and how they should be sealed. Using the services of a family planning clinic, you may not have an opportunity to express these preferences until the day of the operation, when you first meet your urologist.

If you have special needs or preferences about where the surgery takes place, you will have to contact a private urologist. Vasectomies arranged by a family planning clinic are performed on their premises. To determine whether location is an important consideration for you, the next section outlines the three options available.

Choosing a Location for Surgery

The vast majority of vasectomies are safely performed in the urologist's office, and most urologists prefer to do them there. The advantages of having the vasectomy in a urologist's office are convenience and economy, since there is no charge for hospitalization, use of an operating room, or use of a recovery room. The same economies apply in a family planning clinic. The following may be considered disadvantages: in a doctor's office, nothing stronger than a local anesthetic is likely to be administered; few support personnel are available in the rare event of a severe adverse reaction; and most offices don't have an out-of-the-way place for you to lie down if you feel too queasy after the operation to go directly home. However, there is very seldom a need for anything more than a local anesthetic, and after millions of operations there is no indication that office vasectomies are any less safe than hospital or clinic vasectomies.

A private urologist will be affiliated with a nearby hospital, and we think that its outpatient department is an excellent place for your vasectomy. In the outpatient surgery department, the urologist has access to a fully-equipped surgical supply cabinet, additional relaxing drugs should you become excessively anxious, and additional support personnel in case they are needed. And there is a place for you to linger privately until you are feeling better. Having your vasectomy in a hospital outpatient department is more expensive since you must pay a rental fee for the operating room (and a recovery room if you use it), but many medical insurance policies cover these costs.

Your third option, a hospital's major surgery operating room, is the most sophisticated and costly place to have a vasectomy. You should consider it only if you feel certain that you cannot bear to be awake for the two small incisions in your scrotum or if you have a serious heart or other medical condition that requires close monitoring throughout even minor surgery. This means that you will have to pay for a day of hospitalization, the surgeon's fee, the anesthetist's fee, and rental of the operating and recovery room—perhaps as much as $1,000 in all. Most insurance policies do *not* cover vasectomy in a major surgery operating room. If you require or wish this procedure, be certain to check your insurance policy beforehand.

Preoperative Preparation

For any elective surgery such as vasectomy, you should be in the best of health. If you have a cold, flu, or fever, you should postpone the operation. Pimples, boils, or skin diseases of the scrotum should be treated and healed first, and please be sure to bring any of these conditions to your urologist's attention. Left untreated, they can cause complications after surgery.

Avoid heavy drinking or drug use the night before your vasectomy. We feel a little silly giving this advice, but experience has shown that it must be given. Medications given can interact with drugs already in your system to cause an adverse reaction before or during surgery. You should avoid aspirin and aspirin products for a week before vasectomy since aspirin reduces your blood's ability to clot effectively. We would also advise that you take only liquids on the day of surgery. Although it is rare, patients do vomit; with an empty stomach there is no problem.

Your physician will probably ask that you wash your scrotum thoroughly that morning with ordinary soap or an antibacterial soap, such as pHisoHex or Betadine, to lessen the chance of infection. He or she may also ask you to shave your scrotum at home in the shower, where any loose hair is sure to be washed off. Only the hair on the scrotum itself need be removed; hair above the penis can be left alone. Bring a snug-fitting athletic supporter with you to hold the gauze dressings in place as well as reduce your postoperative discomfort.

Part of your preparation for surgery will be mental. It would be surprising if you didn't experience at least a little fear before an operation on your scrotum—or on any part of your body for that matter. Disciples of Sigmund Freud argue that a man's anxiety before a vasectomy relates to a subconscious fear of castration. We think surgery per se is enough to make anyone nervous.

It is possible that your fears of surgery are very intense, strong enough to keep you from having the operation even when you consider it a good idea in every other respect. You may be telling yourself that you should dismiss these fears as childish. But your fears of surgery may be telling you something you are not yet consciously aware of. While strong fears before do not always lead to regrets after a vasectomy, research (Zeigler, 1969) indicates that a man who feels pronounced concern about the impact of vasectomy on his body runs a greater risk of later experiencing postoperative adjustment problems or regrets. If there is any hint that your fear of surgery is related to a deeper fear of long-term effects, we urge you to discuss your feelings with your urologist or counselor.

In all likelihood, your concern about vasectomy surgery falls within the normal range, and you will resolve not to let short-term anxieties interfere with your long-term goal of permanent, effective contraception. We want to stress that anxiety before a vasectomy is normal. You are better off acknowledging your trepidation than pretending indifference to the integrity of your body.

After Your Operation

It is a good idea to have your partner or a friend there to meet you after a vasectomy. You will probably feel a little sore and a little dizzy, and walking more than a block or driving may cause unnecessary discomfort or bleeding.

Go to bed as soon as you get home and place an ice pack over your athletic supporter and dressings for the rest of the day and evening. You should not get out of bed except to get your meals or go to the toilet. Since your testicles are suspended in your scrotum partly by the vasa deferentia, staying in bed and wearing the athletic supporter prevents tugging and reduces the postoperative strain.

When the effects of the local anesthetic have worn off (about an hour or two after the vasectomy), most men experience a dull ache in the testicles and groin. Some men describe it as similar to the feeling that follows a few minutes after being "kicked in the balls." If you wear your athletic supporter, this pain will diminish rapidly in the first day or two. Your surgeon will usually prescribe a mild painkiller such as Tylenol or codeine; by the fourth day, you can switch to aspirin if you still have residual pain. Rarely will you need anything stronger. Very rarely, aching in the testicles will persist for several weeks or months: this type of pain, called chronic orchialgia, is discussed in more detail in Chapter 6.

You can resume sexual activity one week after your vasectomy. You may experience some discomfort in your groin or testicles when you first resume intercourse; this is due to the contractions of the vas deferens that occur during ejaculation. The discomfort will diminish as the internal tissues heal. Full normal

activities including sports and heavy lifting may be
safely resumed two to three weeks after surgery.

In Case of Complications

Every surgical procedure, no matter how minor, carries with it the risk that something can go wrong. Com-
paratively speaking, vasectomy is a low-risk procedure,
and the complications associated with it are usually
easy to control. Most men pass through their surgical
experience and their first week after recovery with
some pain but nothing more. A minority experiences
complications relating to allergies, bleeding, or infection. We want you to know about possible complications.

Occasionally a patient with no previous history of allergies develops a reaction after the injection of local
anesthetic, manifested by an itch and possibly hives.
Very rarely, a patient will develop a more severe reaction, leading to difficult breathing or collapse. Should
this occur, your surgeon will always have medication
on hand to reverse these symptoms immediately.

Some ooze of blood and serum onto the gauze pads is
normal in the first day or two. If the bleeding appears
to be excessive, rapidly soaking the gauze, or if you require more than two or three gauze changes per day,
compress the incision between your thumb and index
finger for five to ten minutes. If this fails to stop the
bleeding, call your surgeon.

Bleeding inside your scrotum may cause a painful
swelling called a hematoma. Hematoma occurs in 0.25
to 4 percent of all vasectomy cases. If rapid swelling of
your scrotum to the size of an orange or a grapefruit
occurs shortly after vasectomy, contact your surgeon
immediately. You may need to have the hematoma

drained. Even if they are stitched together perfectly, the edges of an incision may open up: this is the body's way of letting out blood or pus accumulated inside the scrotum. Once drained, the wound will close itself without any further treatment.

Frequently after vasectomy, some blood may seep between the layers of the skin, giving the scrotum and penis a bruised color. This problem is usually painless and will disappear without treatment in a week or two.

Infection is possible after any surgical procedure but is very rare after vasectomy, occurring less than one percent of the time. If you notice redness, pus, or increased swelling around an incision three days or more after your vasectomy, or if you develop a fever, notify your surgeon. He or she will probably prescribe antibiotics and/or an antimicrobial cream or ointment, in addition to hot baths two or three times a day. Properly treated, infections subside in a few days. If an infection has caused an accumulation of pus, your surgeon may want to open the wound slightly to clean it. Occasionally, a small pimple or abscess will develop near a stitch: this is easily cured by removal of the suture. Infrequently a patient develops an allergic reaction to the suture material used to seal the ends of the vasa: a small knot of inflamed tissue forms inside the scrotum. Again, removal of the offending suture cures this problem.

The most frequent complication after a vasectomy, and a potentially annoying one, is a sperm granuloma, a firm ball of tissue a quarter- to half-inch in diameter, caused by the leakage of sperm from the vasectomy site or from a rupture in the epididymis or rete testis. Such a leak can occur during the surgical process if sperm escape when the vas is cut, or it can occur if the seals

(sutures, clamps, or cautery) on the cut ends of the vas
let go in the first three months after surgery. Later on,
epididymal or rete rupture is the more likely source of
the problem. Granulomas are believed to happen in
anywhere from 30 to 90 percent of all men who have
vasectomies.

Granulomas occur when sperm escape from a leak in
the reproductive tract, provoking an inflammatory
reaction. The body's response to sperm in an abnormal
location is similar to the reaction to an ingrown hair or
nail: it forms a network of pockets and channels that
trap sperm in scar tissue and inflammation cells. If the
nerves of the vas deferens also get trapped in the
granuloma (a relatively rare occurrence), a dull ache
can result. Persistently painful granulomas must be
surgically removed, but most of them are insignificant
and diminish on their own over time. The impact of
granuloma on reversal surgery is discussed in Chapters
6 and 8.

When Are You Sterile?

Your surgeon should emphasize that you will not be
sterile immediately after your vasectomy, perhaps not
for six weeks or more. Mature sperm—in the urethra,
the ejaculatory ducts, and the sections of vasa still connected to those organs—continue in their ordinary
course: it may take several ejaculations before the last
of them are cleared from the "front" portion of your
reproductive system. New sperm being born in the
testes proceed as usual through the epididymis as far as
the seal in the vas, where they are blocked.

After twelve to fifteen ejaculations, or approximately
six weeks, you should go to your surgeon or a medical
lab for a sperm count. In most cases, your surgeon will

give you a specimen bottle and the name of a particular lab. You provide a specimen by masturbating into a bottle, either at the lab or, as many men prefer, at home. You will need to deliver your semen sample to the lab within a few hours after you produce it to insure correct results. Sperm can live outside the human body for only a few hours, so you want to give the technician a chance to see if your sample contains any strongly swimming sperm (a possible sign of spontaneous recanalization).

Approximately three days after you deliver your semen sample to the lab, you should be able to call your doctor or clinic and find out the results. Until the lab confirms that your count is zero, you and your partner should continue to use your current method of contraception. Vasectomies can fail. If a man has more than one vas in his spermatic cord, the doctor may not have discovered it. Occasionally, even a skilled surgeon will mistakenly cut a blood vessel instead of the vas, leaving the patient's sperm delivery system intact. Sometimes, the severed vas will recanalize. *Take no chances. Stay on birth control until the "all clear" is given.*

Vasectomy Failure

True vasectomy failure (as opposed to pregnancy caused by residual sperm in the front portion of the reproductive tract) occurs when live sperm appear in the semen after the normal twelve to fifteen ejaculations. Various studies report vasectomy failure from zero to six percent of the time, with the average being about one percent. Since good results tend to be reported more frequently than bad, the actual failure rate may be somewhat higher than one percent.

Spontaneous Recanalization

By far the most common and frustrating cause of vasectomy failure, spontaneous recanalization, occurs when the two ends of a vas deferens reconnect on their own. The extraordinary capacity of the cells lining the vasa to bore their way through and around ligatures, scar tissue, and steel clips and cross great distances is testimony to the high priority evolution has bestowed upon reproductive functions. Spontaneous recanalization usually occurs after a leak of sperm from the testicular side of the cut vas deferens. The leak results in the formation of a sperm granuloma, a cyst-like nodule that contains multiple interconnecting channels. If one or more of these channels finds its way to the other end of the vas, sperm can move through this alternate route to the front of the reproductive tract. Usually these connecting channels close down from scar formation, but occasionally they stay open and produce vasectomy failure. Fortunately, the majority of spontaneous recanalizations occur soon after vasectomy and can be detected at the first or second postoperative sperm count. However, recanalization has been known to occur after zero-sperm counts have been attained, and as late as seventeen months after vasectomy.

Spontaneous recanalization is possible regardless of the surgical technique used. It has happened even when over two inches of vas were removed from each side. Removal of longer segments can prevent failure, but such a step increases the risk of complications and also makes reversal difficult. Closing both ends of the vas with electrocautery and sealing one end inside the vas sheath with a clip or stitch reduces the failure rate to less than one-half of one percent.

Complications such as hematoma or scrotal infection increase the possibility of failure. Excess scar tissue can form after these complications, pulling the ends of the vas closer together and increasing the likelihood of spontaneous recanalization.

Surgical Error

Although rare, surgical error can cause vasectomy failure. Cutting a structure other than the vas deferens, such as a nerve or blood vessel, occurs less than once in a thousand vasectomies, and it can be detected promptly if a small section of vas is sent to a laboratory for identification.

Even more remote is the possibility that an individual has more than one vas in his sheath. This phenomenon has been detected in less than one in a hundred thousand cases.

What to Do If Your Sperm Count Is Not Zero

If you have had at least fifteen ejaculations and do not have a zero-sperm count, it is possible that you still have some residual sperm hiding in your seminal vesicles or in the abdominal side of the vasa. Have another sperm count done six weeks or a dozen ejaculations later. If moving sperm still appear, this indicates the need for another vasectomy. We suggest that you return to your physician or clinic.

As we have already observed, vasectomy failure almost never occurs after a zero-sperm count has been achieved. Detection of this rare occurrence requires a sperm count one year after vasectomy. Whether you decide to have this "safety check" is an individual decision, best made after discussion with your surgeon.

5
What Are the
Emotional Aftereffects?

In Chapter 3, you encountered some of the emotional challenges that attend the decision-making process. After the operation, similar challenges await you and your partner as you learn to live with the new state of your reproductive system. Needless to say, vasectomy more clearly and directly affects men than women. But a man's vasectomy seems to set off emotions in his partner also, as she comes to terms with the sudden reality that he can no longer make her pregnant. Most of the time, couples respond very well to their new contraceptive freedom.

During the first few months after surgery, a vasectomized man and his partner must invest both time and mental energy in reassessing their self-images and repatterning their relationship. This chapter will take a closer look at that period of reassessment and at some of the changes that are likely to occur, thereby lessening the chance of surprise or potential awkwardness in your postvasectomy experience.

Before moving to the level of individual experience, we'd like to acquaint you with the broad outlines of

some psychological and sociological studies of vasectomized men and their wives (there have been few studies of vasectomized single men). This general background from the social sciences will provide a context
for better understanding the particular aftereffects.

Almost every major study of reactions to vasectomy
has been criticized on one methodological ground or
another (Weist and Janke, 1974), yet it seems indisput-
able that a minimum of 30 percent of couples report
that they have sex more frequently in the first few
months after the operation, enjoy it more, consider
their marriage stronger, feel healthier and more relaxed (this generalization applies especially to women),
and have no regrets about their decision. No more than
12 percent of the men or couples in any of the studies
done in the United States, England, or Canada (other
than those conducted in the psychiatric wards of hospitals) reported any regrets whatsoever about the operation (Wolfers, 1970), and most of those were mild
complaints that faded with time. At least 90 percent of
all men who have had vasectomy say that they would
make the same choice again and that they would
recommend the operation for men in circumstances
similar to their own (Ferber, et al., 1967; Maschhoff, et
al., 1976). Wives seem to feel even more positively
about the operation than the men. Favorable reactions
to vasectomy seem to be distributed uniformly among
younger as well as older couples and among nonpar-
ents as well as parents.

On the other hand, there is a small percentage of
men and women who experience difficulty in adjusting
to male sterilization. Most frequently, their emotional
distress shows up in the form of sexual dysfunction,
such as impotence or premature ejaculation, or gynecological symptoms that make intercourse painful or

impossible. In the worst cases, emotional distress after vasectomy has led to marital crisis or, in a few instances, to mental illness and hospitalization. When the reaction reaches this extreme, vasectomy is probably not so much the cause as a catalyst for an existing problem. These disasters can only be prevented by a thorough evaluation of the couple by their counselor or physician in combination with a rigorously honest self-assessment by the man and the woman.

While the odds are very good that vasectomy will work out well for you, there is a small but noteworthy chance that it will not. Aside from exercising caution as you decide to go ahead with the operation, you can minimize this risk by becoming aware of some of the new and possibly unexpected emotions that may follow in the weeks and months after surgery.

Sex After Vasectomy

Nearly all the men we've spoken to admit they wondered if sex would feel as good after vasectomy. When a man comes home from a vasectomy operation, surely he can't imagine when he'll feel like having sex again. But this condition will pass quickly, and the familiar sexual sensations will reassert themselves. We've recommended that you wait a week after surgery to resume intercourse, but you may be ready for sex somewhat earlier than that—if you adjust the vigor of your lovemaking to the tenderness of your scrotum. The first few times you reach orgasm will bring on some unaccustomed sensations, particularly in your scrotum: your vasa contract as usual during orgasm, but testicular fluid and sperm are building up behind the surgical obstruction for the first time. Again, these new sensations, if they occur at all, are temporary.

Like the men we've spoken to, you may become preoccupied with orgasms in the first few weeks after vasectomy, probably counting them in preparation for your trip to the lab for a sperm count. You may experience a special elation as you get closer to the time when you can throw away those condoms or your partner can leave her diaphragm in the bathroom cabinet. On the other hand, you may find yourself wanting to examine your last ejaculate to discover whether you can see any difference. Sperm are not visible to the naked eye, even when they are present by the millions in your ejaculate.

For many couples, finding out you are sperm-free, that your count is zero, can be an exciting time, one to celebrate with champagne and a flourish, perhaps even a ceremony as you throw your last few condoms into the wastebasket or dump your pills down the sink. Approximately a third of the couples questioned about changes in their sexual patterns after vasectomy reported a one-month to one-year sexual renaissance—renewed interest in sexual intercourse with each other. They attributed their rekindled pleasure in sex to freedom: from fear of pregnancy and from the need to interrupt their lovemaking to fumble with a diaphragm or condom (Weist and Janke, 1974).

Not all couples enjoy so positive a reaction to vasectomy. Some men and women experience a temporary (in some cases a continuing) decline in their sex lives. This group represents a small minority, but their distress can be acute. Since there is no physiological reason for vasectomy to cause impotence or premature ejaculation, these signs of sexual shutdown are almost certainly related to a man's ambivalence or frustration about the vasectomy's meaning in his life. Psychological researchers (Zeigler, et al., 1969) have suggested this explanation of why postvasectomy impotence is a greater problem for older men: almost every vasecto-mized man goes through a period in which he needs to test whether he is still as sexually potent and attractive as he was before the operation, and older men are more likely to overtax their physical capacities by increasing the frequency of intercourse. For the majority of men, successful performance in bed dispels the anxiety, and their sexual patterns return to prevasectomy levels. For a few men, the need to prove their manliness continues to exhaust them sexually and their impotence recurs.

Interviews with men and couples have persuaded us that the major portion of continuing sexual problems are an expression of resentment about the way the deci-sion for vasectomy was reached. Vasectomies elected for symbolic rather than contraceptive reasons and those performed when one partner did not give full and voluntary consent are the most likely to result in un-happiness. For example, a man who submits to a vasec-tomy only because his wife doesn't want another child may later experience a profound anger at having been made "safe" for her. Vasectomy should never mean self-sacrifice, to either partner.

A gynecologist (Fitzgerald, 1972) has treated several women for symptoms that made intercourse painful if not impossible after their husbands decided to have vasectomies without their wives' strong support. Each of these women indicated to Fitzgerald in one way or another that she found sex less worthwhile after her husband was sterilized. Fitzgerald speculated, rightly or wrongly, that there are some women who cannot en-joy sexual relations without the possibility (one could say danger) of pregnancy.

We don't mean to scare you out of having the operation. Rather, we mean only to emphasize the connection between the quality of your prevasectomy decision and the quality of your reaction afterward. Even the small proportion of sexual problems that follow vasectomy can be predicted if the vasectomy candidate, his partner, his surgeon, and his counselor each do a thorough job of exploring the motives for seeking the operation. The prospects are good when all agree positively that vasectomy is the best method of birth control for you.

Do I Seem Different to Others?

Focusing on sexual improvements or declines does not tell the whole story. It appears that men who undergo vasectomy also need to assure themselves that they are not seen as less manly or assertive by the people who are important in their lives—wives or lovers, children, colleagues, and friends. Our experience and interviews confirm the general findings of psychological research into changes in self-image after vasectomy and the impact of those changes on interpersonal behavior: many men seem to go through at least a brief period of self-consciousness, wondering whether anyone is noticing some difference in their masculinity. While this feeling of tentativeness usually lasts only a brief time, it can lead to some nervous tension in the man and those around him. In a few men, problems of masculine image persist and require counseling.

One way to appreciate this self-consciousness is to think about how often or how seldom men you know have told you what form of contraception they are using. Even among close male friends, birth control is apparently a topic that men cannot talk about easily. While natural modesty about their private lives and sexual practices may be at the source of this silence, vasectomy seems to be kept a secret by approximately half the men who have had one (Ferber, et al., 1967), which indicates that they perceive the operation as tainted by a certain stigma that diminishes a man in the eyes of his friends or his family. In the Ferber study, more than ninety percent of the men questioned said they would recommend vasectomy for other men in circumstances similar to their own. When asked if they actually had recommended the operation to anyone else, half admitted they had not; asked why, the men generally replied that relatives and friends would criticize them for committing a sin, becoming less manly, or being overly submissive to their wives.

Postoperative Male Mystique

This concern about the possibility of losing male status in other people's eyes temporarily disturbs approximately forty percent of men who undergo vasectomy (Ferber, 1967; Zeigler, 1971). There is a good chance in the first few months after the surgery that a man will exhibit intensified, somewhat exaggerated masculine behavior. At home he may become reluctant to take on babysitting chores or do the dishes. Children may find their father more likely to impose discipline. Colleagues at work report that these men are more authoritative and decisive. In sum, a recent vasectomy sometimes causes men to become somewhat more "macho."

There is a certain irony here since more than one study (Howard, 1981; Bloom and Houston, 1976; Horenstein and Houston, 1975) has found that men who elect vasectomy tend to be better educated, more open to ideas about the equality of the sexes, and less stereotypic in their masculine attitudes than average.

Apparently even the most enlightened males are vulnerable to the symbolic association with castration and loss of masculine identity.

Intensified male behavior—uneasiness around the kitchen and assertiveness at work—seems to be the analogue of the increased demand for intercourse that is common after vasectomy. In public and in private, he needs to demonstrate that he has lost none of his manly drive.

The Female Reaction

While much more research remains to be done on the topic, it appears that wives for the most part react even more positively to vasectomy than their husbands. Even those wives who are aware that their husbands have become somewhat more sensitive about domestic chores report high degrees of satisfaction with the fact of the operation. Many women seem to thrive on their new-found freedom from the fear of pregnancy, and in one Australian study of couples' reactions to vasectomy, almost half the wives reported an improvement in their overall health. As the researcher put it, "*He* had the operation and *she* felt better!" (Leavesley, 1980).

In first-person accounts of their experience some women recall pangs of guilt about the permanence of vasectomy, regretting their husband's sacrifice to meet immediate contraceptive needs. Many more women, convinced that his decision was made without reservation, consider vasectomy a wonderful gift from a husband or lover who cares about their health, safety, and peace of mind. Statistics on women's satisfaction with their mate's vasectomy are universally better than 95 percent.

As with men, there is a possibility of nonsexual

change that deserves attention. In one study of reactions to vasectomy (Zeigler, et al., 1969), more than a quarter of the wives perceived a decline in the overall quality of their marriage in the year after the operation. The researchers felt that these women found their marriages less satisfying because vasectomy had triggered stereotypic male behavior in their husbands, although the women themselves did not relate the decline in marital satisfaction to vasectomy. Nearly all of them said they were content about their husband's having undergone the operation, perceiving it as a definite benefit to themselves. For the most part, these marriages seem to have returned to preoperative levels of satisfaction within a year or two.

Couples Without Children and Single Men: A Different Set of Reactions?

In Chapter 3, we noted that the emotional issues surrounding vasectomy are essentially the same for couples with or without children. The small amount of research (Brown and Magarick, 1979) on couples without children has thus far identified no emotional aftereffects that do not also apply to couples with children. There seems to be no difference of kind or degree in their postvasectomy experience.

Even fewer studies have been done on single, childless men: the findings indicate that these men take no special risks when they undergo the operation (Denniston, 1978). However, this generalization may be superficial, reflecting research done by questionnaire rather than in-depth interview. Urologists who perform vasectomy reversals observe that a disproportionate percentage of their clients are young, single men, who decided to have a vasectomy impulsively and a few years later changed their minds.

While these impressions about reversal are not scientifically gathered, we do know that men who are single do seem to have some postvasectomy experiences that married, vasectomized men do not. To begin with, a man who has a vasectomy when he is single can obtain his future partner's assent to sterility only after the fact —thus he has the special problem of telling her about his decision to have no children. The data on the general reluctance of men to talk about their vasectomy suggest that this problem may be particularly stressful. A single man, having resolved to confide in his companion, must then cope with uncertainty about her reaction, which can be serious if the relationship is becoming serious. We know that some women break off the relationship immediately because they want (at least eventually) to have a child; others have the opposite reaction, deepening their commitment.

Before having a vasectomy, a single man should confront two certainties; sooner or later he will find himself in a serious relationship, and when he does, he cannot ask for his partner's participation in a decision he has already reached alone. In effect, he may be demanding a sacrifice that he would not demand if present circumstances changed—if he fell in love with a woman who wanted to have children with him. It is appropriate here to emphasize that the majority of requests for vasectomy reversal are made by men who have married recently and who have decided they want a child after all.

Assessing the Emotional Risks

Serious emotional consequences following vasectomy appear to be rare. Most men and women report being more than pleased with the freedom and security vasectomy offers, and both husbands and wives assert that they would make the same choice if they had it to do again. While some researchers have suggested that these couples have a vested interest in defending a decision they cannot unmake, we believe that the reports of satisfaction are too consistent and widespread for massive numbers of men and women to be fooling themselves about the impact of the operation on their lives. As further proof, we would point to the relatively low percentage, somewhere between two and six percent, of men who seek vasectomy reversal and to their reasons for seeking it. Usually these men are not so much dissatisfied with the operation as they are interested in their new marriages, which they wish to consecrate with children.

In a sense, it is misleading to look at vasectomy as a cause of satisfaction or dissatisfaction in a man, woman, or couple. It does not have a power of its own, except to prevent pregnancy. Any *meaning* associated with vasectomy derives from the reasons for choosing the operation in the first place or from the quality of a couple's relationship. Vasectomy can neither save nor destroy a relationship. It can cement a good one or erode a troubled one by focusing both man and woman on their commitment to their future with each other. Similarly, it cannot destroy the self-image of a man whose ego is functioning well, although it can focus him on insecurities that dwell within him already. It cannot make a woman feel less like a woman if she has paid close attention to her feelings before giving her assent. In sum, the potential for unhappy reactions precedes vasectomy. Thus, we would emphasize one final time how important it is to search out this potential before the surgery.

6

What About the Medical Consequences?

For the past several years, the press and electronic media have been reporting that vasectomy might be dangerous to a man's health. Preliminary observations and research findings on both men and animals suggest that vasectomy may be associated with such common afflictions as heart disease, hardening of the arteries (atherosclerosis), blood clotting disorders (thrombophlebitis, pulmonary embolism), kidney disease, and arthritis. In light of the bitter lessons learned from studies of the long-term effects of the Pill, DES, thalidomide, and other reproduction-related medical treatments, reports of potential dangers associated with vasectomy have been taken very seriously by the medical research community and the federal government.

During the 1970s, at least a dozen studies, five of them well-designed and carefully controlled, were launched to determine the medical safety of vasectomy in humans. Their results indicate that vasectomy apparently does not pose a significant risk to a man's overall health. In other words, it does not appear to increase his risk of heart attack, kidney disease, thrombosis, or other serious disorders. Given that approximately thirty million men worldwide have undergone vasectomy, and given that vasectomies have been performed since the 1920s, we can reasonably conclude that medical research would almost certainly have discovered any blatant correlations between vasectomy and a decline in the state of a man's overall health.

This is not to say that vasectomy has absolutely no impact on his body. For example, careful studies have demonstrated that the continued production of sperm, blocked in the vas, generates pressure buildup that can do physical damage to the reproductive system, resulting in minor discomfort in some cases and, on occasion, severe pain. This back pressure can cause tearing or ruptures in the delicate tubules leading from the testicles, a complication that may prevent reversal of the vasectomy.

Vasectomy appears to provoke changes in the immune system of approximately half of all men who have the operation. Composed partly of your white blood cells and lymph, the immune system cleanses foreign substances out of the bloodstream. Science has not yet fully comprehended the complex functioning of the immune system, and the impact of vasectomy on that system is not well understood. It is possible that vasectomy causes a man's immune system to attack and neutralize his own sperm. Occasionally men with this response may not be able to impregnate a woman even after a surgically successful reversal.

Researchers have focused attention on the action of certain immune complexes (antibodies linked to sperm fragments): in rabbits and monkeys these immune complexes cling to the walls of arteries and settle in the kidneys, causing atherosclerosis and kidney disease.

While none of this damage has yet been associated with vasectomy in humans, further research is warranted in this area. For the moment, the only clear risk associated with changes in the immune system is the possibility that they will render a vasectomy reversal futile.

We will be able to take a much closer look at each of the known and suspected side effects after a review of how vasectomy changes the male reproductive system.

How the Reproductive Tract Reacts

Let us begin with what vasectomy does not do. It causes little or no visible change in the testicles or scrotum. The tiny scars and any discoloration disappear in a few weeks. The seminal vesicles and prostate continue to produce seminal fluids, and thus a man's ejaculate will look the same to him as before the operation. Vasectomy has no noticeable impact on testosterone or other hormonal outputs.

Vasectomy may affect production of sperm in the testes. Studies of dogs (Lepow and Crozier, 1979) show that new sperm leaving the epididymis build up at the vasectomy site, causing pressure which slows the production of sperm. In humans, this pressure is never transmitted all the way back to the testes. Instead, testicular fluid and sperm are absorbed and evacuated in the vas deferens, the epididymis, and the rete testis. Some of the pressure may also be attenuated by formation of a granuloma, a cyst-like knot that increases the amount of tissue surface available for absorption of pent up sperm. Thus little disruption of the sperm-producing function of the testes occurs in humans. Biopsies up to fifteen years after vasectomy show the testes to be normal. At worst, vasectomy may slow the rate of sperm production in some men, but their sperm production rate seems to return to normal after a reversal.

Because the pressure buildup in the system bears most directly upon the delicate tubules of the epididymis and the rete testis, these channels can become swollen and tense after vasectomy. In about one percent of the cases epididymal congestion with sperm and fluid becomes painful, causing a condition called chronic orchialgia. Usually this dull ache in the testes disappears in three to six months. In perhaps one out of a hundred thousand men, chronic orchialgia must be relieved by vasectomy reversal or unsealing the testicular end of the vas.

Sometimes one of the tiny epididymal or rete tubules will rupture from the pressure of sperm backup. Sperm leak from the point of the rupture, causing either a sperm granuloma or a blockage of the duct. This is of little consequence unless the individual later seeks a reversal, since a damaged or blocked rete or epididymis makes restoring fertility less likely.

Vasectomy also causes some changes in the vas deferens. While the outside of the vas remains the same, the inner opening (called the lumen) usually becomes much wider after a vasectomy, indicating that some of the muscular tissue surrounding the lumen has deteriorated. While the widening of the lumen is painless and usually of no consequence, it too may contribute to disappointment if a man decides to attempt vasectomy reversal; the muscular tissue left in the repaired vas may not be sufficient to push sperm along its length. Loss of contraction in the muscles of the vas deferens can also result during surgery from inadvertent damage to the blood vessels and nerves located in the surrounding sheath.

Sperm Granuloma

Although granulomas may occur in up to ninety percent of all vasectomized men, most granulomas have no significant adverse effects. As we noted in Chapter 4, however, if one of the sperm-laden channels in a granuloma connects with the ejaculatory, or front, side of the vas, the system can reconnect itself and result in vasectomy failure.

With regard to the long-term consequences of a sperm granuloma, it represents both a potential asset and liability for the vasectomized male. Evidence in animals and humans suggests that a granuloma protects the epididymis and rete testis from some of the damage of built-up pressure after vasectomy (Silber, 1977). The granuloma acts like a valve in a steam pipe, venting some of the pressure by providing extra surface area for the absorption of fluids and dead sperm. Sherman Silber, M.D., has concluded from his experience performing vasectomy reversals that a sperm granuloma on the testicular end of a divided vas enhances the likelihood that the vas can successfully be reconnected.

On the negative side, a sperm granuloma seems to increase the likelihood that a man's immune system will form antibodies against his own sperm. Since these antibodies may have other significant consequences, and since they may be formed by processes other than the appearance of sperm granulomas, let us further explore the topic of antibodies against sperm in the next section.

Antibody Formation and Immune Reactions After Vasectomy

To understand the complex biochemical reactions that occur after vasectomy, we must first answer the question of what happens to the sperm that continue to be produced in the testes and absorbed in the rete, the epididymis, and the vas. After vasectomy, a balance develops between sperm production and breakdown. Production probably slows down, and the epididymis and vas adapt to absorb much more testicular fluid and "digested" sperm. After vasectomy, sperm are broken down in the vas and epididymis into their chemical components, which then dissolve harmlessly in the surrounding fluid. In turn, this fluid is absorbed and carried away in the body's blood and lymph fluids. However, some of the sperm in the vas as well as most of the sperm in granulomas do not get completely broken down and dissolved. These undissolved pieces of sperm may stimulate the formation of antibodies when they get into the bloodstream.

Antibodies Against Sperm

Antibodies are the foot soldiers of the immune system, the body's general defense network against infection and disease. The immune system has the uncanny ability to distinguish between those chemicals and cells that are normally present in the human body and those that are foreign, such as viruses, bacteria, and toxins. If such an agent should slip past the body's external defenses, the immune system's cells will recognize the breach and start making specific defender cells, antibodies, to neutralize the offending agent.

Normally, the immune system does not attack tissues or cells that have been in your body since birth. Unlike other cells, sperm do not appear in a man's body until puberty, and they have specialized surface characteristics that make them targets for recognition as foreign by the immune surveillance system. Ordinarily, sperm or parts of sperm never come in contact with immune detectors; in the testes they are segregated behind a barrier of cells, and during transport through the epididymis, vas, and urethra they continue to be shielded from direct contact with blood cells or lymph fluid. Antibodies against sperm are rare in nonvasectomized men. If, however, this self-contained system is violated by vasectomy or any operation or injury that allows sperm to leak outside the barrier, antibodies directed against sperm can form in the blood.

As we have already mentioned, some experts hypothesize that antibodies against sperm can prevent the return of fertility even after the vasa deferentia have been surgically reconnected (Linnet, et al., 1981). By causing large numbers of sperm to clump together or immobilize, antibodies can render them unable to swim successfully through a woman's reproductive tract. After a successful reversal, antibody levels usually drop or disappear entirely from the bloodstream.

Some medical researchers believe that the phenomenon of antibody formation is connected to disease in men who have had vasectomies. Antibodies against sperm often combine with sperm fragments and circulate in the bloodstream in aggregates called immune complexes. Usually, immune complexes are cleared quickly from the blood and rendered harmless, but an immune complex will sometimes stick to a blood vessel wall, joint surface, or kidney causing damage. It has been suggested that immune complexes sticking to a blood vessel may attract deposits of cholesterol and fatty substances called plaque that could cause atherosclerosis.

The Evidence on Circulatory Aftereffects
The first reports of circulatory difficulties that might be related to vasectomy were published in 1971 by H. J.

Roberts, M.D., who observed a disproportionate number of cases of thrombophlebitis and pulmonary embolism in vasectomized men. These men were all heavy
smokers, but Roberts suspected that their blood vessel
and clotting disorders were related to anti-sperm immune complexes in the circulatory system. Subsequent
studies of large numbers of men failed to confirm Dr.
Roberts' suspicions, though they increased interest in
the search for possible long-term effects of vasectomy.

One of these studies is being conducted by Dr. Nancy
Alexander and colleagues at the Oregon Primate Research Laboratory. Dr. Alexander has found a significant increase in hardening of the arteries among
vasectomized monkeys, especially those fed a high-cho-
lesterol diet (Alexander and Henderson, 1979; Clarkson
and Alexander, 1980). This small, well-controlled study
has raised some questions about the safety of vasectomy in humans: data derived from studies on monkeys
will raise more attention than those on rats, rabbits, or
guinea pigs. However, species differences are often significant in reproductive research, and monkeys are not
strictly comparable to the human male. Furthermore,
monkeys living in cages experience very different envi-
ronmental stresses than do humans. Neverthless Dr.
Alexander's provocative reports have stimulated investigation of the potential for heart or blood vessel aftereffects in man.

Five of these studies (Walker, et al., 1981a; 1981b;
Verheugt, et al., 1981; Wallace, et al., 1981; Bullock, et
al., 1977) employed matched controls: in other words,
the long-term medical histories of vasectomized men
were compared to those of nonvasectomized men of
similar age and health. The Walker study examined the
records of over 6,000 men and found no significant differences in hospitalization rates. A second comparison

of 4,830 men by Walker and his co-researchers found no increase in heart attacks.

There is no good evidence at present that these antibodies cause disease in humans. If there is a link between vasectomy and disease, it is likely to appear in the form of a correlation with hardening of the arteries. Dr. Alexander has identified a marked increase in hardening of the arteries of vasectomized cynomolgus monkeys on a high cholesterol diet. A smaller increase was also detected in vasectomized monkeys eating regular food. Dr. Alexander has speculated that this damage to the blood vessels is due to immune mechanisms. These observations suggest that an extensive study of the effects of vasectomy in humans is warranted. To date, however, no diseases or chemical abnormalities other than anti-sperm antibodies have been found in men after vasectomy. No excess deaths from blood vessel, heart, or immune diseases have shown up. If vasectomy does pose a risk to man, then it must be small.

Are the Medical Risks Acceptable?

The early reports on the medical safety of vasectomy indicate that the risk of any serious aftereffects is low. The millions of vasectomies performed and the few good studies presently available virtually eliminate the possibility of disastrous consequences like those traced to thalidomide and DES. A strict, detailed comparison between vasectomy and other widely used forms of contraception as to health effects is not available at this time because very large, long-term studies (like the ones that identified the risks of the Pill) are still in progress. The studies by Dr. Alexander and her colleagues are legitimate cause for concern: it is possible that vasectomy involves a risk for hardening of the arteries in man. Perhaps vasectomy, like the Pill, will be a less desirable contraceptive choice for those who expose themselves to other risk factors such as smoking, obesity, or a sedentary lifestyle. We will have to wait at least ten years for results from the long-term studies to answer these questions. As of this writing, it seems that the medical consequences of vasectomy are not serious. But it is clear that possible risks, known and unknown, must be weighed against advantages when making any contraceptive choice. In the next chapter, we will examine some of those other available choices.

7
A Comparison of the Birth Control Alternatives

You now have a comprehensive picture of the advantages and disadvantages of choosing vasectomy as your method of contraception. On the positive side: barring recanalization during the first few months, a vasectomy virtually guarantees effective birth control for the rest of your life, requiring no further contraceptive efforts on your part; it will not interfere with your pleasure or spontaneity during sexual intercourse; and it is less expensive than female sterilization or long-term use of the Pill. The disadvantages of vasectomy include possible but as-yet-undiscovered long-term physical side effects, especially if you have a tendency toward high blood pressure, atherosclerosis, or heart disease; potential stress or anxiety induced by the operation's symbolic challenge to your sense of manhood; likely conflict between you and your present or future partner if you are not in agreement about the advisability or necessity of the operation; and changes in the epididymis and other parts of your sperm delivery system that may lower your chances of restoring fertility at a later date.

Of course, the terms "advantage" and "disadvantage" are comparative rather than absolute. To place vasectomy's benefits and risks in perspective, the operation must be compared against the benefits and risks of the other means of birth control currently available to you and your partner. No contraceptive is perfect, by which we mean both completely effective and completely free from adverse side effects. Among the nonpermanent methods of contraception, the general rule is the more effective it is in preventing pregnancy, the more likely it is to cause side effects; less risk of dangerous side effects means less protection against accidental pregnancy.

Still there is a large array of contraceptive alternatives, each with its advantages and disadvantages, and you should consider all of them before deciding that vasectomy, or any other method, is best for you. We have grouped them into four categories: female sterilization (tubal ligation and hysterectomy); effective, nonsurgical female birth control (the Pill, IUD or intrauterine device, and diaphragm); less effective methods (gels, foams, and creams); and male birth control (the condom and coitus interruptus). It is conspicuous, and perhaps significant, that three of the four categories consist of female-centered measures. Regrettably, the only method known that involves active cooperation of both man and woman is rhythm, and still more regrettably, it may be the least effective. In light of the fact that both authors are men, we have tried to set forth the available alternatives, male and female, with as much sensitivity and objectivity as possible in the short space of this chapter. If you wish more detailed information, we recommend a talk with your physician or family planning counselor.

Female Sterilization

Tubal Ligation

Vasectomy's only strict equivalent for the female is tubal ligation, surgical interruption of the fallopian tubes. By blocking the channels that carry eggs from the ovaries, tubal ligation prevents conception from taking place. Some women refer to the procedure as "having their tubes tied," but this image is misleading. With a tubal ligation the fallopian tubes, like the vasa deferentia during a vasectomy, are actually severed, after which they are tied, clamped, banded or electrocauterized. Even with modern microsurgical techniques, success rates in reversing tubal ligation run around 30 percent, much less than the average for successful vasectomy reversal.

There are four methods for performing tubal ligation: laparotomy, laparoscopy, colpotomy, and culdoscopy. Most physicians consider the laparotomy the safest form of tubal ligation. The laparotomy is performed by making a relatively small incision in the lower abdomen, locating, grasping, and ligating the fallopian tubes, and then sealing and returning them to the abdomen. By contrast, laparoscopy employs two small incisions, one on the lower abdomen, one higher up near the navel. Air is pumped in to inflate the abdomen. Using a remarkable combination light-and-microscope called the laparoscope, the surgeon locates the fallopian tubes, cuts and seals them, and then closes the incisions after the air has been removed and the laparoscope withdrawn. Both colpotomy and culdoscopy involve locating the fallopian tubes through an incision made in the vagina. This approach is less preferred in the United States, Canada, and Western Europe than are laparotomy or laparoscopy.

The advantages of tubal sterilization are basically those of vasectomy: if no recanalization occurs, tubal ligation is permanent and requires no further concern about contraceptive measures. Also, it is relatively inexpensive, requiring only an overnight stay in the hospital. Unlike vasectomy, tubal ligation is not known to cause any immunological changes in the body.

However, it has certain disadvantages when compared to vasectomy. Complication rates for tubal ligation are definitely higher; serious potential complications after a laparotomy or laparoscopy include hemorrhage, heart arrhythmia, bowel perforation, infection, and severe pain. Because both laparotomy and laparoscopy involve opening the abdomen, these operations have a small but definable statistical risk of complications that can lead to the patient's death, once in every 100,000 cases. There is good evidence that tubal ligation increases the chance of an ectopic pregnancy, a pregnancy that occurs in a fallopian tube rather than the uterus. Ectopic pregnancies always require surgery, often require the removal of the fallopian tube, and must be detected in time to save the patient's life (Ticker, 1981). Surgical failure and recanalization occur once in every 200 cases. Failure and complication rates for laparoscopy are higher than laparotomy, while vaginal methods appear to have the highest failure rate of the three.

In the emotional realm, tubal ligation can pose the same problems of adjustment to sudden sterility that occur in recently vasectomized men. Like hysterectomy and menopause, tubal ligation has been known to precipitate an "empty womb syndrome" in some women (Barglow, 1964). In these cases the permanence of the operation, perceived beforehand as a source of security, afterward becomes a source of guilt. Self-esteem drops and depression follows. The fear of having become less feminine or less completely a woman after sterilization usually disappears quickly, but the self-doubt can be uncomfortable to live with for a while and may require counseling or psychotherapy if it persists.

In practice, tubal ligation reversal is even more difficult to achieve than vasectomy reversal. The rate of success may be lower because fewer gynecologists who perform ligation attempt to preserve the maximum amount of fallopian tube. Some gynecologists tend to remove or destroy several inches of tube in order to lower the chance of spontaneous reconnection. However, as women begin to insist on a minimum of tubal removal, and as the number of requests for reversal increases, there is every reason to believe that the success rate in ligation reversal should approach that of vasectomy reversal. Of course, requesting that a minimal segment of the fallopian tubes be removed brings with it a higher risk of recanalization, and the desire to retain improved chances of successful reversal should be weighed against the desire for failure-proof sterilization. There is also an increased risk of ectopic pregnancy after reversal in women.

Vasectomy or Tubal Ligation?

Vasectomy has several apparent advantages over tubal ligation: usually it does not involve a stay in the hospital, it is less expensive by $300 to $500, less likely to provoke medical complications, and more likely to be reversed successfully. From a medical viewpoint, it is probably less risky for a man to have a vasectomy than for a woman to have one or another form of tubal ligation. However, a sterilization decision is most frequently a decision about the nature of a couple's relationship rather than a series of technical judgments about the safety or cost of a particular form of surgery. Only rarely are all things truly equal. In our opinion, neither vasectomy nor tubal ligation is risky from a medical point of view, and the difference in cost is hardly enough to tip the balance. Except in cases where one or the other member of a couple simply cannot undergo surgery, we recommend that the decision be based on the process outlined in Chapter 3. Sterilization of either partner involves too many emotional vulnerabilities and too many chances for later regret to let a thousand dollars or two nights in the hospital determine your choice.

Hysterectomy

A trend toward hysterectomy—the surgical removal of the uterus, or both uterus and ovaries—simply for birth control purposes has begun to appear in the United States. Gynecologists who support this practice say that once a woman has decided she wants no more children, the uterus and ovaries are no longer necessary and their removal can reduce the statistical chances of breast cancer and other gynecological diseases. We feel, however, that hysterectomy should not be performed for birth control purposes, because tubal ligation at least allows the possibility of surgical reversal if a woman changes her mind about not wanting additional children. Furthermore, hysterectomy is major surgery with a noticeably higher risk of complications than tubal ligation, and six times the mortality rate. In our view, hysterectomy should be performed as a response to existing or impending disease; as a mere birth control measure, it is too drastic.

Nonsurgical Female Birth Control

Only three other means of female birth control approximate the reliability of tubal ligation or vasectomy: the Pill, the IUD, and the diaphragm. While the Pill is almost as reliable as sterilization, it appears to be less safe from a medical standpoint, particularly for smokers and women in their thirties and beyond. The IUD is almost as effective as the Pill, but it seems to have some medical dangers of its own. The diaphragm appears to be safer than sterilization, though it is far less effective. For those women or couples who are not yet ready for the permanence of male or female sterilization, the Pill, IUD, and diaphragm represent the best available alternatives.

The Pill

The Pill is the popular name for tablets that inhibit ovulation. It has been controversial since its introduction in the early 1960s and is likely to remain so for the foreseeable future. Government studies from the late 1960s indicate that prolonged use of the Pill increases the chance of thromboembolism, a clotting disorder that can cause stroke, thrombophlebitis, and death. In addition, the Pill is associated with an increased risk of myocardial infarction (heart attack). Both of these risks are increased in women who smoke. As we noted in Chapter 1, the increase in the number of vasectomies in the early 1970s can be correlated with the news that the Pill might pose a hazard to a woman's health. In recent years, hormonal levels in the Pill have been reduced and reformulated so that it is safer for general use, but concern about the Pill's long-term effects still remains.

When first marketed in the 1960s, the Pill contained high levels of synthetic female hormones that prevent ovulation if administered in sufficient quantity. Currently, most versions of the Pill have lowered levels of these hormones, which seems to moderate the side effects. Still, one woman in four experiences side effects such as nausea, suppressed menstrual bleeding, fluid retention, breast enlargement, headache, spotting, weight gain, and breakthrough bleeding, that is, bleeding at mid-cycle.

Aside from the minor side effects associated with menstruation, there is a potential for more serious medical complications. For example, the Pill has been known to alter the liver function in a small percentage of women; women suffering from hepatitis, mononucleosis, or other liver disorders should not take the Pill, at least until those conditions clear up. The Pill is known to cause gallstones in 70 out of every 100,000 users who would not otherwise have developed the problem if they were not taking the Pill. Gallstones can be very painful and sometimes require surgical removal. For women who are already susceptible to diabetes, the Pill can hasten its onset—although the Pill does not by itself seem to cause diabetes. It can also cause a slight rise in blood pressure; women with hypertensive disorders, a susceptibility to heart disease, stroke, or migraine should not be on the Pill. Finally, the Pill can cause increased susceptibility to vaginitis and venereal disease, trigger depression, and suppress a woman's sexual desire (Roberts, 1979).

The most common serious complication that arises from use of the Pill is thromboembolism, or circulating blood clots. Thromboembolism can be a dangerous, even life-threatening condition if a blood clot lodges in the heart, lung, or brain. The Pill appears to cause thromboembolism in a small but still significant number of women who would not otherwise have contracted the condition. Among all women between the ages of twenty and thirty-four, one in 500,000 dies of thromboembolism; among Pill users in the same age group, the rate climbs to nearly eight in 500,000. Among women thirty-five to forty-four who do not use the Pill, 2.5 in 500,000 dies of thromboembolism; among Pill users, twenty in every 500,000. To put this risk in perspective, we should note that among all pregnant women 100 in 500,000 succumb to thromboembolism; in that sense, pregnancy is more dangerous than the Pill (Tucker, 1981).

Recently, reports indicate that Pill-taking may slightly increase a woman's chance of suffering a heart attack, perhaps as much as two to fourfold. These risks appear to be increased even more in smokers. At present, researchers believe that this risk may persist, particularly in smokers, even after they have stopped taking the Pill (Stadel, 1981).

The Pill seems to present no other life-threatening risks to a woman. Despite the addition of hormones into the bloodstream, there have been no studies as yet that implicate the Pill in breast or other forms of cancer. To be on the safe side, however, women who suffer from benign tumors of the breast, as well as those who have already had cancer of the reproductive system, should avoid the Pill.

Having understood and weighed the potential for harmful side effects, we can consider the effectiveness of the Pill: it is usually described as more than 99 percent effective under ideal conditions, which means the woman conscientiously takes her pills on schedule. If taken conscientiously, less than one user in 100 will become pregnant each year; the actual rate is probably

closer to two or three per 100. Most of these pregnancies result from forgetting to take the Pill as prescribed.
Some women become pregnant while on the Pill simply because every method of contraception, including
sterilization, sometimes fails. While the Pill has a
higher failure rate than a correctly performed male or
female sterilization, it has the lowest failure rate of all
nonsurgical methods of contraception.

Vasectomy or the Pill?

The Pill is not without its risks: we will know more
about them, such as the link with heart disease, as
more results of long-term studies come in. So far the
Pill probably represents the best alternative for younger women and couples who are looking for highly effective, nonpermanent contraception. For women over
the age of thirty-five, the risk of thromboembolism and
heart attack may be excessive, and in most cases these
women should consider some other birth control alternative, especially if they are smokers. The only nonsurgical alternatives that approach the effectiveness of the
Pill are the IUD and the diaphragm.

IUDs, or Intrauterine Devices

An IUD is a small piece of plastic, manufactured in
one or another coiled shape, that is implanted in the
uterus. Attached to its base is a plastic thread that
trails through the cervix into the vagina. We do not
know precisely why they work, but some IUDs seem to
work better when wrapped in a copper thread. While
the IUD is not as effective as the Pill, it is less risky for
older women and has fewer side effects. In the course of
a year, between 2 and 4 percent of women using the
IUD will become pregnant. A great majority of these
failures occur among women who have never had a

child or have used the IUD for less than one year. Like a vasectomy or tubal ligation, an IUD does not inhibit spontaneity during lovemaking.

A gynecologist can insert an IUD in even less time than it takes a urologist to perform an office vasectomy. After performing an internal exam, the physician dilates the cervix and carefully places the IUD in the uterus. The gynecologist must make certain that the thread hangs down through the cervix and into the vagina, as the presence of the thread in the vagina is the means by which a woman can tell if her IUD is still in place. Having an IUD inserted may cause a day or two of cramps, like severe menstrual cramps. Normally these subside. However, many women report that their menstrual cramps are more severe and their bleeding heavier as long as the IUD remains in place. These uncomfortable changes are probably caused by the efforts of the body to expel the IUD as it is shedding the lining of the uterus.

When an IUD fails, it is usually because the woman's body rejects and expels the device. IUD rejection most often occurs within the first year and most often coincides with menstruation, when a woman is less likely to notice that the IUD is gone. An IUD user should check for its presence at least once a day by locating the thread leading into her vagina. If she cannot find it, she should contact her gynecologist at once.

Recent reports indicate that the IUD may be more dangerous than was believed only a few years ago. An IUD can perforate the uterus, allowing the device to pass into the abdomen; a runaway IUD must be removed through surgery. Another risk is infection: if the IUD picks up bacteria from the vagina and conveys them to the uterus, the patient can develop pelvic inflammatory disease (PID), which must be treated with heavy doses of antibiotics. The risk of PID in IUD users is 1.7 times as great as those not using contraception. PID has been known to create adhesions around the fallopian tubes that can make subsequent pregnancy impossible. IUDs can cause inflammation of the uterus, sometimes requiring removal of the device. They can also cause tubal or ovarian abscesses. In 5 to 10 percent of IUD failures, the pregnancy will be ectopic, and 30 to 50 percent of IUD failures result in spontaneous abortion if the IUD is left in place (Rosenfield, 1978).

Vasectomy or the IUD?

The far greater risk of complications and the far higher rate of failure make the IUD not strictly comparable to vasectomy. As a temporary form of birth control, the IUD has some advantages to offer as a meaningful alternative to sterilization: it is easier to have an IUD inserted than to have a vasectomy and usually less expensive; if it is working well, the copper IUD requires replacing only at three-year intervals, and the plastic IUD not at all, depending on your doctor's preference; and the IUD does not interfere before, during, or after intercourse.

While there is a chance of uterine damage, PID, and ectopic pregnancy, there is no known hormonal or immunological risk whatsoever associated with an IUD. Another factor to consider is that some gynecologists recommend abortion if a woman becomes pregnant while her IUD is in place because of the possibility of spontaneous abortion. Most gynecologists recommend removing the IUD which can also result in spontaneous abortion.

Diaphragms

Because they appear to be virtually free of any negative side effects or medical risks, diaphragms have been making a strong comeback among women and couples seeking safe, nonpermanent contraception. Reports indicate that each year 2 to 17 percent of diaphragm users become pregnant, but further research has shown that many of these pregnancies happen because of improper insertion, failure to use the recommended creams or jellies with the diaphragm, or laziness on the part of the user rather than because of some technical flaw in diaphragms as a birth control device (Hatcher, et al., 1976). For women who are conscientious about using it, the diaphragm can be a highly successful and completely safe form of nonsurgical birth control.

The main drawbacks relate to the work involved in using a diaphragm. It must be washed, powdered, and stored as a matter of routine. A woman may have to interrupt her lovemaking to insert the diaphragm, although many couples integrate diaphragm insertion into their foreplay, and it can be inserted up to four hours prior to intercourse. A woman who uses a diaphragm must place a spoonful of spermicidal gel into it before insertion and then feel around to make certain that the diaphragm is properly placed over her cervix and behind her pelvic bone. While the diaphragm has no medical or hormonal dangers associated with it, not every woman is willing or able to spend this much time and attention on the practice of contraception.

If you are motivated to use it properly, a diaphragm can be worthwhile. A doctor measures and fits you for a diaphragm in a single visit, and when inserted, it should create absolutely no discomfort. Though it cannot match sterilization in preventing pregnancy, the diaphragm does represent a safe and reasonably effective alternative for individuals and couples who are not yet ready for permanent birth control.

Gels, Foams, Creams, and Suppositories

Because these methods are so much less effective than sterilization, the Pill, the IUD, or the diaphragm, Table 7–1 says nearly all that needs to be said about spermicidal gels, foams, creams, and suppositories. It should be noted that there is now some concern among scientists that spermicidal substances may be associated with somewhat higher rates of birth defects.

Table 7–1

Method	Percent of Failure Under Ideal Conditions
Vasectomy	0.1
Tubal ligation	0.1
Pill	0.5 – 2
IUD	2 – 5
Condom	4 – 10
Diaphragm	3 – 17
Rhythm	13 – 21
Gels, foams, creams	14 – 22
No contraception	60 – 80

Sources: R.A. Hatcher, et al., *Contraceptive Technology, 1976–1977* (New York: Irvington Publishers, 1976) and Fork, K., "Contraceptive Efficiency Among Married Women 15–44 Years of Age in the United States, 1970–1973," *Advancedata* 26 (1978):2.

Male Birth Control

There are basically three forms of male contraception other than vasectomy: condoms, premature withdrawal (coitus interruptus), and abstinence timed for when a woman is likely to be ovulating. This last, the rhythm method, is more properly thought of as shared responsibility for contraception. However, all of these methods are so ineffective that using any of them for five or ten years with a normal frequency of intercourse almost guarantees at least one accidental pregnancy in a fertile couple.

Condoms

Among the male-centered, nonsurgical forms of birth control, condoms are probably the most popular and effective, despite their reported annual failure rate of 4 to 10 percent. A condom is a thin rubber or animal-skin sheath that prevents sperm from entering a woman's vagina and thus prevents conception—if the condom stays on, doesn't leak, and isn't put on too late. A recent study (Free and Alexander, 1976) indicates that men who are highly motivated to use a condom properly have relatively good success preventing pregnancies (only one percent attributable to the failure of the condom itself, rather than failure of the man to use the condom). Some men have learned to include putting on a condom in their foreplay, and some will tell you that condoms improve lovemaking by prolonging the time it takes them to reach ejaculation; others complain that the condom interferes with their sensual enjoyment of intercourse. Condoms have the health advantage of being completely safe and offering some protection from venereal diseases.

Choosing the condom as a means of contraception relates to the choice for vasectomy in two possibly significant ways. First, vasectomy candidates use condoms more frequently than men in the general population. Thus, a man who seeks vasectomy is more likely than the average to have been taking responsibility for contraception. This ethical or psychological orientation may shed some additional light on whether the man or

the woman in a relationship is a better candidate for
sterilization (Howard, 1981).

Second, studies have shown that at least one-fourth
of the men who seek vasectomy have been involved in
one or more unplanned pregnancies, and some of these
men were using a condom. It is possible that a contraceptive failure when the male is taking responsibility for birth control may lead to a hasty conclusion that
vasectomy is the inevitable alternative. If this scenario
seems to apply in your relationship, we would advise
you to explore with your partner and a counselor why
you do not wish to try out nonpermanent forms of
female birth control before taking the step of permanent sterilization.

Coitus Interruptus and Rhythm

Coitus interruptus is easily the least effective means
of birth control, one whose failure rate approaches the
use of no contraceptive whatsoever. There is a good
reason for this method to fail; a man's urge to remain
in the vagina at the time of orgasm, as well as the practical difficulty of timing withdrawal. The first and
most powerful spurt of a man's ejaculate contains most
of the sperm, and even a split second can be much too
late to prevent conception.

Rhythm seems to have a somewhat better record
than premature withdrawal. Motivated couples can
form an estimate as to when the woman has ovulated
by counting the days from her last period, taking her
temperature and checking the thickness of the cervical
mucus (the Billings method). Even scrupulous calcu-
lations and conscientious abstinence during the estimated time of ovulation eventually prove ineffective
because sperm can live in the uterus for several days.
While rhythm is becoming more popular because it is

completely safe hormonally and immunologically, its use over several years virtually guarantees an unplanned pregnancy in a fertile couple.

Vasectomy Compared Overall

Vasectomy, then, seems to have a number of advantages over all other means of birth control. It is the most effective, except for total abstinence. Once a man has a vasectomy, he and his partner never have to think about or plan contraception. A vasectomy is relatively easy to perform and inexpensive, and it does not require a long recovery period in most cases. There are few clear medical risks associated with vasectomy, and it is usually manageable from a psychological or emotional perspective. Of the female-centered methods that approach vasectomy in effectiveness, none can be said to be as safe, and none of the very safe measures, such as the diaphragm, condom, and rhythm, is nearly as effective.

Nevertheless we feel compelled to leave the subject of vasectomy and tubal ligation with a reminder that they differ radically from all other forms of birth control, not so much because they are highly effective but because they are permanent. Ultimately, the greatest risk of sterilization is that you will change your mind. Your chances for successful reversal are somewhat better than even.

In the next chapter, we will examine the remarkable advances in microsurgery that make vasectomy reversal possible; then we will look at the psychological dimensions of trying for reversal and coping with its success or its failure.

8
The Miracle of Microsurgical Reversal

Since the 1970s, the number of American men who undergo vasectomy has stabilized at 400,000 to 500,000 annually. By contrast, the number requesting surgical reversal of vasectomy has grown dramatically. Ten years ago, most experts estimated that in the United States the annual number of requests for reversal equaled less than one percent of all vasectomies performed, perhaps one reversal for every thousand vasectomies. Current estimates range from 2 to 6 percent (Fenster and McLoughlin, 1981): thus, each year, between 10,000 and 30,000 American males seek to have their vasa deferentia surgically reconnected.

In Chapter 3, we urged our readers to consider vasectomy as permanent and to request the operation only if they were certain that their decision would hold, regardless of any change in personal or family circumstances. This chapter should make it abundantly clear that a reversal is not a simple matter, so we must stand by our recommendation. Nevertheless, time undermines the best intentions and clearest resolutions, and we recognize that increasing numbers of men and couples have valid reasons for considering reversal: a new marriage, the death of a child, dramatically changed economic circumstances, or a simple change of heart about a decision made during an earlier, more impressionable time of life. This chapter will also cover the practical aspects that become important when you are deciding whether to try for reversal, such as hospital costs, insurance, and choice of surgeon, in addition to offering certain guidelines to help you evaluate and maximize your chances for success.

As we have mentioned, under the best of circumstances, conventional reversal techniques lead to pregnancy less than 50 percent of the time. However, spectacular advances made in microsurgery since the mid-1970s hold out even more hope that thousands of men will be able to restore their fertility. A cautious attitude in approaching vasectomy and guarded optimism in approaching reversal are still desirable, yet microsurgical techniques and the growing skills and experience of the surgeons who use them are shifting the balance in favor of the man who changes his mind.

The Evolution of Vasectomy Reversal

Since vasectomy was not practiced before the twentieth century, the history of vasectomy reversal is brief, the first report appearing in a medical journal in 1931. Early attempts at reversal were crude by contemporary standards: while quantities of sperm appeared in the ejaculate of reversal patients, pregnancy rates reached a mere 5 to 35 percent.

It is not difficult to understand why these early results were poor. As we noted in Chapter 2, the vas is only as thick as a venetian blind cord, about 2/10ths of an inch, but that is the outside diameter. The inner channel through which the sperm travel is only 1/100th of an inch in diameter, virtually invisible to the naked eye. For a reversal operation to be successful, this tiny inner opening must be accurately reconnected to allow the free flow of sperm. The first experimenters simply stitched the outer diameter of one end of the vas to the other, with no attempt to align the inner lumen.

When the problem of inner alignment became apparent in the 1950s and 1960s, few techniques or materials were yet available to solve it. Some experimenters inserted thread, wire, or tubing in both ends of the lumen to keep them lined up and then sewed the outside diameter of the vas over this splint, which would later be removed. Unfortunately, the splint either irritated the lining of the vas or left a hole after its removal, after causing a sperm granuloma to form, blocking the flow of sperm. Other methods of reconnecting the lumen openings, such as stitching them side-to-side or end-to-side, proved equally unsuccessful. Surgeons were still working with relatively thick suture material, and without magnification. Reversing a vasectomy under these circumstances is about like stitching a garden hose with coarse hemp and a needle as thick as a pencil. You wanted no leaks and perfect alignment, but you could use only three or four stitches. To comprehend the added difficulty of working on structures almost too small to see, imagine sewing that garden hose in a dark room.

Just as the invention of the microscope opened new aspects of the world to scientists over three centuries ago, the development and application of special microscopes vastly expanded the horizons of modern surgery. The use of the microscope in human surgery dates back to 1921, when it revolutionized operations on the inner ear. In the 1950s, eye surgeons using the

microscope achieved better results with delicate operations on the cornea and retina. Although the magnification afforded by the microscope allowed better
visualization of tiny structures, the lack of suitably
small needles and sutures held back further development of microsurgery.

By the 1960s, manufacturers of surgical equipment
were producing needles 1/250th of an inch in diameter
(thinner than a human hair) and sutures as fine as
1/1000th of an inch in diameter (invisible to the naked
eye). With the new technology came the need for new
skills: surgeons had to learn to sew while peering
through the eye pieces of a microscope using a specially
adapted jeweler's forceps or tweezers. After hundreds
of hours practicing on animals, the first microsurgeons
performed previously impossible feats, such as repair-
ing nerves and blood vessels 1/100th of an inch in size
and removing tiny tumors deep in the brain.

In 1968, urologists employed microsurgical techniques to perform vasectomy reversals in dogs. Using
conventional techniques, success had been attained
only 8 percent of the time. With microsurgical techniques, success jumped to an astounding 95 percent. In
the mid-1970s, Sherman Silber, M.D., a St. Louis urologist who spent several years in the laboratory trying
out microsurgical procedures on rats, applied his skills
and experience to human vasectomy reversal. In the
first years of his efforts, Silber reported a 71 percent
pregnancy rate (Silber, 1977). Shortly thereafter, Earl
Owen, M.D., a skilled Australian microsurgeon, reported similar results (Owen, 1977). Silber's current
pregnancy rate of 82 percent, in couples followed
at least 5 years, is truly remarkable. Controlled com-
parisons against conventional techniques confirm the
clear superiority of microsurgical vasectomy reversal

(Thomas, et al., 1979), (Fenster and McLoughlin, 1981), (Lee and McLoughlin, 1980), (Hampel, 1978).

Choosing a Microsurgeon

By contrast to vasectomy, vasovasostomy is a difficult and lengthy operation, requiring a stay in the hospital and considerable skill on the part of the surgeon. Accurate reconnection is probably the single most important factor determining whether sperm will reappear in your ejaculate. There is no margin for error. Accordingly, the best results are obtained by the most-practiced urologic microsurgeons, those who perform the operation frequently.

You should seek a surgeon who uses an operating microscope for the procedure, has had animal laboratory training in microsurgery, and devotes a significant portion of his or her practice to microsurgical procedures. Since there are only a handful of skilled microsurgeons in this country who perform vasectomy reversal, finding one will often necessitate travel to a major medical center. The best sources for such referrals would be the urology or microsurgery departments of the university's medical center or

The American Fertility Society
1608 13th Ave. South, Suite 101
Birmingham, AL 35256

Association for Voluntary Sterilization, Inc.
122 E. 42nd St.
New York, NY 10168

American Society of Andrology
c/o Dr. Howard R. Nankin, M.D.
University of South Carolina Dept. of Medicine
V. A. Hospital, Bldg. 28
Columbia, SC 29208

You may have to wait several months for a surgical appointment, particularly since vasovasostomy is an elective procedure and receives lower priority in hospital operating rooms than emergency cases or operations to combat disease. But a truly skilled urologic microsurgeon is well worth the wait.

A Word about Costs

Taking into account the surgeon's fee for a difficult operation, the anesthesiologist's fee, the rental of the operating room, the charge for staying at the hospital, and any expenses you might incur traveling to a major city to find an experienced urological microsurgeon, you may find vasectomy reversal an expensive proposition. It is common for the procedure to total anywhere from $4,000 to $8,000. Should you have to remain in the hospital longer than planned, costs can run well beyond that. Some but not all insurance companies cover varying portions of this total. It is wise to check with your insurance company in advance before making a surgical appointment.

What to Expect During Microsurgical Reversal

Because there are more variables than in vasectomy, it is not possible to describe the "typical" reversal operation; surgery can last from two to six hours (three seems to be the average), and the procedures that a urologic microsurgeon will use are determined in large part by what he or she finds once the scrotum has been opened. In some cases, only the two severed ends of the vas need to be reconnected. This procedure is known as a vasovasostomy. But sometimes damage to one or both epididymi will make it necessary for the surgeon to perform a vasoepididymostomy, a connection of a vas end with the epididymis beyond the site of the damage, closer to the testicle. Vasoepididymostomy usually takes longer than vasovasostomy, and places an even greater premium of the skill of the microsurgeon.

There is no reliable technique that enables a surgeon to know ahead of time precisely what operation he will have to perform. This can only be determined at the time of surgery.

Because you will require major anesthesia for a reversal attempt and because you should lie quietly for a day or two after surgery, we suggest that you have your reversal operation in a hospital. While occasionally a sophisticated outpatient facility may meet the requirements of reversal, usually only a hospital operating room is equipped with the necessary microscopes, anesthesiology, and staff. One key member of the operating team is the pathologist or technician who, as the operation progresses, rapidly examines samples of vas fluid to determine whether sperm are present.

Your preparation for the reversal operation is exactly the same as that described in Chapter 4 for vasectomy. Your surgeon will give instructions as to when to check into the hospital and how long prior to surgery to stop eating. All your scrotal and groin hair will need to be shaved; if your surgery is scheduled in a hospital, an orderly will usually do this for you.

You will have a choice of anesthetic: spinal, which permits you to stay awake without experiencing any pain; or full anesthetic, which puts you to sleep during surgery. Because even a two-hour operation can be a very tedious experience for the patient, most urologic microsurgeons suggest that their patients accept full anesthesia.

Once you have been placed on the operating table

and the anesthetic has taken effect, the surgeon will make a one-inch vertical incision on one side of your scrotum and identify the sealed ends of your vas. If only a small piece of vas was removed at the time of the vasectomy, the ends will usually be close together, perhaps connected by scar tissue. If a long piece of vas was removed, it may be necessary to extend the scrotal incision into the groin or abdomen to obtain enough vas to close the gap. Once both ends of the vas have been identified and freed up (see Figure 8–1), the surgeon will cut across the end of the vas that leads to the ejaculatory duct, passing a fine thread into its opening or injecting fluid to make certain that the channel is open and clear all the way to the urethra.

A cut across the scarred end of the other section of vas, leading to the epididymis and testicle, produces a gush of testicular fluid if there is no other blockage further up. The pathologist examines a sample of this fluid under the microscope to determine if sperm are present. If no fluid flows from this cut, or if sperm are not present in the fluid, the surgeon makes successive cuts further back on the vas until he reaches fluid containing sperm.

If some years have passed since the vasectomy, the surgeon may have to cut all the way back to the epididymis before fluid containing sperm appears. The longer the interval since your vasectomy, the more likely it is that pressure buildup can cause a rupture in the walls of the epididymis or rete testis; the rupture, in turn, can cause leakage of sperm and the formation of a granuloma.

If there has been damage, the surgeon will have to perform a vasoepididymostomy, connecting the vas end to the epididymis somewhere above the point of rupture. A vasoepididymostomy is much more difficult

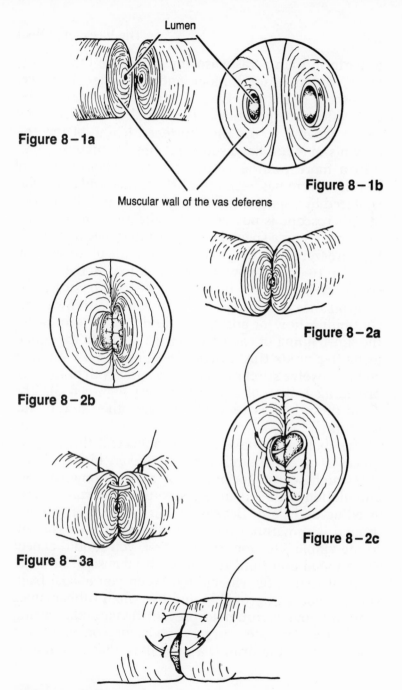

Lumen

Figure 8 – 1a

Figure 8 – 1b

Muscular wall of the vas deferens

Figure 8 – 2a

Figure 8 – 2b

Figure 8 – 2c

Figure 8 – 3a

Figure 8 – 3b

to perform than a vasovasostomy because the walls of the epididymis are thinner and its lumen narrower than those of the vas. Even if surgically successful, reconnection at a point near the testicles can mean that sperm moving across the shortened length of the epididymis may not have sufficient time to mature.

In a more routine vasovasostomy, when a flow of healthy sperm has been established, each end of the vas is placed in a special stabilizing clamp, and the operating microscope is positioned for the anastomosis (connection). Using a special electric cautery needle held by fine tweezers, the surgeon staunches all bleeding: Under the 16- to 40-power magnification of the microscope, even a single drop of blood can obstruct the surgeon's view. While fine jets of water wash away the continuing flow of spermatic fluid, the surgeon sews the inner lining of each section of the vas to the other, using five or six tiny stitches (see Figure 8–2). Another eight to twelve stitches secure the outer wall of the vas, providing leakproof connection (see Figure 8–3). The same procedure is repeated on the other side of the scrotum.

After both vasa have been reconnected, the surgeon makes a careful search for any broken blood vessels that might cause formation of a hematoma, an accumulation of blood in the scrotum that can lead to swelling and pain. Because a fair amount of groping around is sometimes required to free up the vasa and locate viable sites for reconnection, you should expect more blood and fluid to leak from your scrotum after reversal than after vasectomy. When you awake from surgery, you will probably find two small rubber tubes draining your scrotum to prevent hematoma. During a visit the day after surgery, your surgeon will most likely remove the drains, a procedure that is painless.

Your scrotum will be swathed in gauze pads held in place by a scrotal supporter.

Typically, reversal patients leave the hospital after a day or two. We suggest that you bring a jogging suit or some other loose-fitting pants to go home in. The discomfort you are likely to feel after reversal surgery is similar to that after vasectomy (see Chapter 4). However, if your operation required vasoepididymostomy or an incision into the groin or abdomen, the pain is likely to last longer and be more intense. Postoperative care and instructions are exactly the same as for post-vasectomy recovery. You can expect the oozing to last a few more days than it did after vasectomy, and you should consider wearing your supporter for a longer period of time. To minimize any possibility that the delicate reconnections might pull apart, we recommend that you plan to take a week off from work and avoid any heavy lifting or sports for two or three weeks. You may resume sexual activity in one to two weeks, depending upon your surgeon's assessment and advice.

As for the cosmetic aspects, reversal scars will be longer and more noticeable than vasectomy scars.

Potential Complications

Again, the potential complications are essentially the same as after vasectomy. Perhaps the major exception to this generalization is hematoma, which occurs more commonly after reversal. Even with the utmost care in sealing all the tiny blood vessels and the insertion of drains, it is not possible to prevent hematoma in every case. If you develop a severe hematoma while in the hospital, your stay may have to be extended for a day or more. You will probably only want to lie in bed, take painkillers, or take warm baths, as each of these helps to ease the discomfort.

Sperm granuloma, which is again a common side effect of vasectomy, is considerably more disturbing after reversal. A granuloma is a mass of sperm cells and scar tissue that builds up around a leak from the vas or epididymis. Its presence at the site of a reversal indicates that the connection has leaked. The blockage or inflammation that results is almost certain to prevent sperm from passing through the reanastomized vas. On occasion a granuloma can become painful and require surgical removal.

Steps to Restored Fertility

If the operation is a success, the reproductive system begins a gradual recovery after reversal. A swollen epididymis will return to its normal size, and testicular production of sperm, which seems to diminish somewhat after vasectomy, returns to its prevasectomy levels. The return of full sperm production in the testes does not guarantee a return to prevasectomy sperm levels in the ejaculate; most experts agree that even the best sperm counts after reversal are only two-thirds of what they were before vasectomy. This could be due to damaged epididymi, lost transport ability in the vasa, scarring down of the anastomoses, or rarely antisperm antibodies on your semen.

Your surgeon will probably ask you to have a sperm count every month or two until a pregnancy occurs and at least once a year thereafter. The time it takes to achieve pregnancy varies considerably.

Pregnancies often do occur within three to six months after reversal, but typically occur between 6 months and a year. We should emphasize, however, that numerous pregnancies have been recorded two to five years or more after reversal. Our recommendation is that you and your partner begin trying to conceive as soon as comfort permits: If you were ready to go through with a reversal, you should be ready for a pregnancy any time it happens.

In some cases, sperm counts begin to drop slowly during the second and third years after reversal. If your count remains persistently low or near zero for a year or more, the time has come to consider a second operation. While your surgeon will make it clear that success is never guaranteed, it should be noted that second or third attempts are often successful and that failure after one attempt should not be considered a hopeless situation.

Predicting Success or Failure

Two criteria determine the ultimate success of a reversal: the return of sperm to the ejaculate and pregnancy. As we noted above, the first does not guarantee the second. A reversal sometimes produces good sperm counts and motility rates but no pregnancy for several reasons: incompatibility between sperm and the vaginal fluids of the female; female infertility; sexual problems between the partners; and so forth. If we assume that the female verified her fertility before the reversal, that the male verified his before vasectomy, there are several signs that appear during the operation that can help predict whether your fertility is likely to be restored.

Generally, the interval of time between the vasectomy and the vasovasectomy does influence success rates. As a rule, the longer the interval the greater the likelihood that damage has occurred to the epididymi, necessitating the more difficult vasoepididymostomy. Under such circumstances pregnancy rates will be 10–15 percent lower. Dr. Silber (1978b) has shown that after surgically successful reversal, the odds of regaining at least a low-range normal sperm count exceed 90 percent if the vasectomy is less than ten years old; after ten years the odds drop to 59 percent.

Obviously the condition of the vas relates to the difficulty of the vasectomy reversal. We have already indicated that having a minimum amount of vas removed during vasectomy significantly facilitates reversal surgery. Another consideration is whether the vasectomy was performed on the straight portion of your vas, where the segments are easiest to reconnect, or in the convoluted portion near the epididymis, where accurate reconnection is more difficult.

Paradoxically, granuloma can also provide a clue. Though it can lead to the failure of either a vasectomy or a reversal, the presence of a granuloma at the vasectomy site prior to reversal can often be a sign that your reversal has a better-than-average chance of succeeding. As we indicated in Chapter 6, a granuloma at the cut end of the vas can promote recanalization, but it also serves as a safety valve, allowing spermatic fluid to escape and relieving back pressure that can damage the vas and epididymis. Dr. Silber (1977b) has concluded that the presence of a granuloma at the vasectomy site correlates with distinctly higher rates of success in his reversal operations.

Dr. Silber has also conclusively demonstrated that analysis of testicular fluid taken during the reversal procedure is of great value in predicting whether a reversal attempt will succeed. When sperm appear normal or the fluid is clear, the prognosis is usually very good. If no sperm or mostly damaged sperm are found, the outlook is considerably less optimistic. When your surgeon visits after the operation, ask about the analysis done on the testicular fluid.

Only at the time of your reversal operation can the surgeon judge whether conditions in your case are encouraging. A 60 to 80 percent success rate is possible in the hands of a skilled urologic microsurgeon. But remember that the outcome is uncertain in every case, however promising, until an adequate sperm count and pregnancy are achieved. Coping with the uncertainty must be figured into your decision to seek reversal. The next chapter previews the emotional aspects of this decision, which is as significant and even more challenging for a couple than the decision for vasectomy.

9
Is Reversal
Right for You?

Reversal is a gamble, sometimes exhilarating for a couple but sometimes painful. Both the reversal decision and its outcome demand deeper emotional commitment than vasectomy. With vasectomy, the result is virtually assured—the male will become sterile—and the great majority of couples reports complete satisfaction with its impact on their relationship. In the case of reversal, each partner must be willing to risk failure, live with ambiguity, and assume the responsibilities brought on by success. This chapter will help you explore some of the issues that require examination before you undertake vasectomy reversal. It will also try to help you anticipate some of the emotional responses that attend eventual success or failure and to suggest ways of surviving the time inbetween, when neither outcome has yet become apparent. First, let us look at some of the people who seek reversal and examine some of their reasons for seeking it.

Typical Reversal Candidates

The profiles of typical vasectomy candidates, drawn in Chapter 3, show some interesting changes by the time reversal is under consideration. While single men account for a fair number of the vasectomies performed, the decision to try for reversal almost always takes place in the context of a marriage—very often a second marriage for one or both partners. With vasectomy, the man and his partner usually have had at least one child together, but couples who seek reversal usually have not, and often the female has never had children. American women are marrying later now, and many postpone childbearing until after thirty. A significant number of these women marry a divorced man with children from his earlier marriage: in this context, a reversal can be loaded with meaning and peril as the couple tries to build a new marriage and integrate his children into a new family. For the man, it involves renouncing a vow that he would never, regardless of circumstances, change his family. His previous children may well resent the alteration in his feelings. His partner faces trying to become pregnant and carrying and delivering a child at an age when the risks are greater. And both of them have to deal with the possibility that they will not be able to have children together, since reversal attempts fail almost as often as they succeed.

Single men who have vasectomies and later marry, as well as intentionally childless couples who have a change of heart, represent a small but significant portion of those who request vasovasostomy. The heightened social and political consciousness of the 1960s led some young people to request sterilization because they were truly concerned about the population explosion or the state of a hostile world. Since the end of the Vietnam War and the marked decline of birth rates in the West, these reasons are now rarely given for sterilization requests. However, concerned young men who underwent vasectomy during the 1960s are often candidates for reversal today.

In developed countries, divorce is the most common reason for reversal, whereas the death of a child is the most common in developing countries, where infant mortality rates are high and divorce rates low. Still, many couples in the United States seek sterilization reversal after the tragic death of a child. Dr. Sherman Silber, for example, has performed a double reversal for a remarried couple—both a tubal reanastomosis and a vasectomy reversal—after the husband's son by his previous marriage was killed in an accident. The couple was not only able to conceive a child but went on to have another.

Occasionally, a man will request vasovasostomy because he is experiencing a health problem—physical weakness, mood changes, and decreased sex drive— that he believes is directly attributable to his vasectomy. While these symptoms indicate that the patient would benefit from counseling, reversal surgery may well turn out to be the only means by which he will obtain relief. Of course, the counseling alternative should be pursued before the surgical.

Finally, a simple change of heart is not an uncommon and entirely valid reason for requesting reversal. Couples who chose sterilization years before can legitimately decide to have children or more children. Observers such as Gail Sheehy and Roger Gould have alerted us to continuing change as an essential part of adulthood, just as it is a part of childhood and adolescence. An individual's goals, values, and lifestyle may and often do evolve significantly, and if such changes affect decisions about parenthood, it should not be surprising.

As the number of requests for reversal increases, urologists have been gathering an impressionistic but consistent picture of the typical couple seeking reversal. Some of their observations are revealing. Most frequently, the male has children but the female does not. She is likely to be the one who first raises the question of vasectomy reversal: this pattern has made many urologists suspect that older men sometimes submit grudgingly to vasovasostomy merely to please a new wife, though they remain indifferent about its outcome or secretly hope it fails. The opposite situation can also happen: a new wife may assent to her husband's sterilization reversal, not because she wants a child, but because he has expressed his wishes strongly.

As with most of the emotional dimensions of vasovasostomy, the full range of motives has barely been mapped, and much more remains to be known about the couples who seek the operation. Reversal deserves more attention from psychological researchers. If it seems possible that either you or your partner harbors ambivalence about sterilization reversal, we urge you to consult our List of Counseling Services for help with your decision-making process.

Coping With the Likelihood of Infertility

Before undertaking surgery, your urologist will probably want to have some indication that both of you are likely to be fertile. Men who are childless usually have no way of knowing whether they were fertile before vasectomy, since it is not routine to have a sperm count before the operation. In such a case, there may be an examination to determine whether there is any organic reason for the patient to be infertile, followed by a sperm count—just to make certain that the vasectomy has not already spontaneously recanalized without the patient's knowledge.

If the female partner has ever been pregnant, has regular menstrual periods, is less than thirty-five years old, and is in reasonably good health, she is very probably fertile. If, however, the female partner has a prior history of infertility, she should undergo a thorough gynecological exam before a reversal attempt.

Once you've decided that you want to go ahead with a reversal, you've taken the first step on a long journey through the valley of uncertainty. In the United States, one couple in six who are trying to conceive has an infertility problem. While most infertile couples never expect to have difficulty, the reversal couple volunteers for their frustrations. A reversal couple can never know just how long their inability to conceive will last. If months or possibly years pass with sperm counts below normal, a couple might begin to blame each other for their bad luck. Each time the female gets her period, representing one more failure, both she and her partner can slip into melancholy and anger. Ultimately, they may regret that they ever let themselves hope for a child together. Or they may share a wonderful excitement when the male's sperm returns to his ejaculate, and both can take special satisfaction when conception finally occurs. One thing is certain: neither of you will ever take the reproductive process for granted again.

Monitoring Sperm Counts

As we mentioned in the previous chapter, sperm may not appear in a man's ejaculate for three or more months after surgery. Your surgeon may ask you to have your ejaculate tested every month or two, and the process can be burdensome. The sample must be examined under a microscope within the first hour after you produce it to determine the motility of your sperm, their ability to swim strongly in a straight line. In addition to counting the number of sperm per milliliter of ejaculate, the laboratory technician will also calculate how many are damaged, fragmented, or clumped together. Your surgeon may also want to know the pH balance of your semen. Unfortunately, the typical neighborhood medical laboratory is not equipped to perform a postreversal semen analysis, and you will have to go to a major hospital or clinic laboratory.

While you can produce a sample at home and deliver it to the lab in a clean container, it is probably best to produce one at the lab itself. After you have masturbated into a specimen bottle, you notify the receptionist or a technician that your semen sample needs an immediate reading for motility. After going through this process a few times, most men seem to lose interest in finding out exactly how their sperm counts are doing. While some urologists interpret this as evidence that the man is not highly motivated and perhaps never really wished for the reversal to succeed, it is easy enough to understand why a man would avoid this somewhat unappealing routine. Bearing with the discomfiture is probably worthwhile in the long run, as it may eliminate at least one area of uncertainty. Uncertainty is a major source of stress and conflict during the months or years of waiting for conception.

Don't be surprised if the first results are disappointing, even negative. Most fertility specialists consider that pregnancy rarely occurs with fewer than 20 million sperm per milliliter of semen and motility of less than 50 percent. More likely than not, it will take a reversal patient several months before his count reaches even these low-range normal levels. Most counts attain their maximum one year after the operation, though it is not unusual for reversal patients to have counts such as 10 million sperm per milliliter with 40 percent motility at that time. Pregnancies can certainly occur on counts as low as this, but the odds are against quick results. These ambiguous counts, if they do not improve over the course of months, can be harder to live with than the outright failure of a reversal attempt.

The main reason that most reversal couples are unable to conceive a child is the male's inadequate or barely adequate sperm count. There are other factors that may prevent conception or add months to the time it takes. In most reversal couples, both partners are over thirty years old: a woman's fertility drops noticeably after that age. Furthermore, since most reversal couples have not had children together, there is no certainty that they would ever have been able to produce a child, even if each of them has had children in another relationship. Sometimes the acid content of a woman's vagina renders sperm unable to penetrate the cervix. Her body may have an immune reaction that immobilizes his sperm. Or his body may have the immune reaction: almost half of vasectomized men develop antibodies against their own sperm. Sometimes older couples do not have sex frequently enough to guarantee conception. And among couples young or old, part of the problem might be the pressure felt by the man to perform sexually on the schedule of his partner's ovulation.

There are several things that a postreversal couple can and should do to maximize their chances for conception, particularly since it is likely that at best the man will regain only low-range normal sperm counts. The couple should consider the services of a hospital or private fertility clinic. An andrologist monitors the male partner's progress toward normal sperm counts, while the female's ability to conceive is enhanced through a gynecologist's careful assessment of her diet, smoking and drinking habits, metabolic functions, and gynecological health. The clinic will also have staff members who specialize in counseling couples who are facing the unique marital problems that infertility can create.

If you are not ready to seek medical advice from a fertility clinic, there are some things you can do for yourself. In the bibliography, we have listed some good books on infertility and how to overcome it, and we particularly recommend Dr. Silber's *How to Get Pregnant*. All of these books will explain how to identify when ovulation occurs so that you can have intercourse at the most likely time for conception. The couple should abstain for three days prior to the projected ovulation so that the man's ejaculate will contain the maximum quantity of sperm. Abstinence for more than three days adds very little advantage. Since the first spurt of ejaculate contains the highest concentration of sperm, having intercourse a second time soon afterward probably hinders conception somewhat, diluting the concentration of sperm with additional seminal fluid. The conventional male-on-top position promotes exposure of the cervix to the ejaculate. Also, the female should not stand up after her partner's ejaculation for twenty minutes or so in order to allow the sperm enough time for penetration.

Stepping Up from Failure

In the previous chapter, we briefly explained the main indication of reversal failure: a sperm count of zero or near-zero. In some cases, sperm never reappear in the ejaculate. Repeat operations in such cases usually reveal that scarring or granuloma closed the vasa soon after the first reversal surgery. However, most reversal failures are not immediately apparent: some sperm return to the ejaculate for a while. For this reason, we recommend that a reversal couple try to conceive as soon as the male can resume intercourse. Because sperm counts are so unpredictable after reversal, the couple may have only a few months or as much as a year in which to succeed. Many normally fertile couples try to plan conception in the most "convenient" month; reversal couples should not indulge themselves in this luxury.

If sperm counts drop to zero or motility becomes nil because of vas blockage, a couple must decide whether to try a second operation. We have heard of one determined man who has undergone five reversal attempts, each one of which produced a painful hematoma but no offspring; most people would not be willing to undergo both the emotional and physical stress of such persistence.

There are alternatives to a second vasovasostomy. Adoption is attractive to some couples, particularly those who have already given birth to natural children of their own. In cases where the female has never given birth to a child, some couples turn to artificial insemination with sperm from an anonymous donor. This can be a difficult choice if the man feels ambivalence about seeing his wife pregnant but not by his own sperm. If the man's count is close to normal with good motility, there is a third option: sperm banking. Several samples of his ejaculate are collected at a lab and centrifuged to concentrate his sperm. The sperm are frozen and stored until his partner is ovulating. Then a concentrated dose of his sperm is placed directly on her cervix to maximize the possibility of conception. Your surgeon will have to advise you whether your counts and motility are high enough to justify this effort. The general topic of sperm banking will be discussed in the next chapter in greater detail.

Some Closing Thoughts on Reversal

Throughout this chapter, we have adopted a conservative stance on the prospects and problems of reversal. We wanted to give you a realistic introduction to the emotional pitfalls because investing your hopes in this process takes courage, patience, and faith in each other. We do not mean to discourage you from choosing reversal. We only want you to remember that the whole purpose of the operation is to contribute to your relationship, and you may have to work hard at not letting it have the opposite effect. Optimism has a way of turning into bitterness if we are not prepared for disappointment.

Despite the experiences of hematoma, failure, repeat operations, and disappointment, we still favor reversal, one of us as doctor, one as patient. For a man, reversal can mean renewed harmony between his passions and the life-giving forces within him. It can create a binding empathy in a new relationship or restore the sense of commitment in a long-standing one. Men testify to feeling a special relationship to their children born after a reversal, just as the involvement in surgery, recovery, and renewed fertility has given them a special kind of identity with their partner in the creation of life. If you decide to take the exhilarating gamble of reversal, we wish you luck, success, and happiness—and all the healthy babies you want.

10
The Future of Male Birth Control

The increasing number of requests for microsurgical reversal indicates a growing need for improved forms of nonpermanent male birth control. A survey done at the urology clinic of King's College Hospital in London revealed that 40 percent of the men who sought vasectomy there would actually have preferred some form of a male Pill if only such an alternative existed (Reading, et al., 1980). As we have already noted in Chapter 7, current forms of nonsurgical male birth control are neither highly effective nor convenient, at least in the next few years, and they are not likely to be improved significantly in the search for a nonpermanent alternative. The absence of sperm in a man's ejaculate is a far better guarantee against conception than diversion of ejaculated sperm. Improvements in vasectomy reversal will bring us closer to the ideal, but we are still waiting for the male Pill, a 100 percent reversible method that prevents the development or the ejaculation of mature sperm.

While the news media occasionally report the possibility of a major research breakthrough, the truth is that no safe, highly effective, easy-to-use male contraceptive is yet on the horizon. In response to the problems that developed when the Pill and thalidomide were rushed into the market, the Food and Drug Administration (FDA) has made it more time-consuming and expensive to develop and test contraceptives and other drugs related to human reproduction. Quite rightly, the agency fears that a new drug or hormone will cause genetic damage. By the most conservative estimate, the time needed to develop and safety-check a male Pill is at least ten years, and the cost is bound to exceed $50 million. With these constraints, it is unlikely that a commercial pharmaceutical company will try to develop a new male contraceptive in the near future.

However, research into male contraception has been going on at universities and private foundations, focusing mainly on three stages of the male reproductive process: sperm production, sperm maturation, and sperm transport. Such things as hormone injections that suppress sperm production or maturation, chemical agents that perform the same task, valves that temporarily close the vasa, and other techniques do hold some promise for the future. Thus far, each of these experimental techniques has shown unacceptably high failure rates or harmful side effects in humans. But these approaches to more effective temporary male contraception may point the way for the long-term future. We would not recommend that a man considering vasectomy cancel his surgery and wait until these methods are perfected; we thought the reader might be interested to know what the next generation of male birth control techniques will probably look like.

Interfering with Sperm Production

Science still has a number of things to learn about how the male reproductive system works, but certain of the basic chemical and hormonal functions and relationships are well understood. We know that the male hormone testosterone is produced by the Leydig cells of the testes and circulated throughout the body to maintain an adult male's secondary sexual characteristics and his sex drive. Testosterone, along with the pituitary hormone FSH, also stimulates sperm production in the seminiferous tubules. The amount of testosterone produced in the Leydig cells is controlled by a glandular network that includes the testes, anterior pituitary gland, and hypothalamus. Through a feedback system, each of these glands reads the hormonal output of the other two and adjusts its own production accordingly. The testes produce testosterone only if signaled by the pituitary gland, which releases LH and FSH, luteinizing hormone and follicle stimulating hormone. Together, LH and FSH stimulate testosterone output and sperm production. In a sense, the pituitary is like a thermostat, reading the level of testosterone in the bloodstream: if it is too low, the pituitary secretes LH and FSH, and testosterone production increases; if the level is too high, the pituitary lowers its output of LH and FSH, and testosterone production slows down.

The pituitary does not govern alone. Its ability to secrete LH and FSH is regulated by LH-RH, LH-releasing hormone, which comes from the hypothalamus, a gland that sits at the base of the brain. When the hypothalamus detects an insufficient level of LH in the bloodstream, it restores the balance by releasing LH-RH, which stimulates the pituitary to release LH and

FSH, which in turn stimulate the testes to release testosterone and generate sperm.

With an understanding of how this glandular network functions, you can see that suppression of spermatogenesis in the human male should be possible in any of several ways. If the testes could be persuaded not to produce testosterone, the seminiferous tubules would not be stimulated to produce sperm. If the pituitary gland could be stopped from producing LH or FSH, the testes would have no signal to produce testosterone and sperm. If the hypothalamus could be stopped from releasing LH-RH, the pituitary would not release LH or FSH, and eventually production of testosterone and then sperm would cease.

Chemicals and hormones that disrupt the network already exist, but they have several risks, the most significant being potential genetic damage. If a hormone or chemical is attacking a man's reproductive system while sperm are being formed and genetically encoded, there is a chance they will suffer mutation. If the chemical or hormonal contraceptive fails and the man remains partially or completely fertile, the damage to the sperm may produce birth defects. To avoid this risk, some researchers advocate contraceptives that do not affect sperm as they form but arrest sperm as they mature. However, all the chemical and hormonal substances known to cause infertility in men also cause toxic side effects. While the benefits are obvious, the risks are formidable.

Chemical Agents
Recently, chemical methods to shut down sperm production have been prominent in the news. Scientists in the People's Republic of China report that gossypol,

derived from cottonseed, suppresses spermatogenesis after sixty to ninety days of regular use, and that when the drug is discontinued spermatogenesis resumes soon afterward with no sign of genetic damage or diminished fertility (Djerassi, 1981). While there is no question that men who take gossypol soon have markedly diminished numbers of sperm in their ejaculate, scientists are uncertain whether this happens because sperm are no longer being produced or because, as the Chinese claim, they are destroyed in the epididymis. The Chinese claim a 99 percent success rate in temporary sterility with gossypol.

When news of the Chinese breakthrough first reached the West, it was greeted with great excitement. Cottonseed is very inexpensive and widely available here. However, research in the United States and elsewhere indicates that gossypol robs the body of potassium and thus may cause liver damage in man. Taken in large doses, gossypol has also been found to cause fluid in the lungs, shortness of breath, and paralysis (Steinberger, 1971). Testing and approval of gossypol will take many years and millions of dollars. If gossypol itself proves unsatisfactory, chemists may still be able to synthesize a gossypol-like substance that has its contraceptive effectiveness without toxic side effects.

Other chemical agents such as the antibiotic nitrofuran, the dinitropyrroles, and the indol-carboxylic acids suppress sperm production, but they too have dangerous side effects if taken in the dosages necessary to produce near-zero sperm counts. *Bis*-dichlorocetyl is very effective as a sperm repressor and apparently less toxic than the others mentioned above, but it has one inconvenient and unpleasant side effect: if taken in conjunction with alcohol, *bis*-dichlorocetyl causes nausea and vomiting.

Hormone Injections

In the long run, hormones may hold more promise than chemicals. Unusually high levels of various male hormones (androgens) in a man's bloodstream can "fool" the pituitary gland into halting production of testosterone in the testes. Without a direct supply of testosterone, the seminiferous tubules will not generate new sperm. Male hormones administered into the bloodstream maintain the secondary sex character-istics, but, because of the barrier of cells in the seminif-erous tubules, do not reach high enough levels to stimulate sperm production. The injected hormones do however affect the pituitary gland, which interprets the higher level of androgens as a signal that the testes are producing too much testosterone. As the pituitary low-ers its output of LH and FSH, testosterone production in the testes diminishes and spermatogenesis ceases. When the androgen injections are halted, LH and FSH production returns to normal and fertility returns in three to twelve months. Ideally, injections of androgens of one sort or another should be the functional equiva-lent of the Pill.

In reality, things are not so simple. Androgens in pill form are not absorbed well into the bloodstream, so a man must either visit his doctor's office every two weeks to receive his injection or, like a diabetic, learn to inject himself. Any laziness or lapse of memory can lead very quickly to partial restoration of fertility. A sperm count of less than 10 million per milliliter of ejaculate, which is very low, is often sufficient to cause pregnancy. The question of partial fertility has become crucial since experiments have shown that even mas-sive doses of androgens do not necessarily produce azoospermia, the complete absence of sperm. The most successful experiments report zero-sperm counts in no more than 90 percent of the men treated (Barfield, et al., 1979). This success rate is equal to or below that of the condom, which has none of the potential side effects of hormone injections. There is reason to believe that androgen injections over a long period can lead to prostate cancer, heart disease, kidney damage, and metabolic disorders. Unless researchers can synthesize significantly more effective androgens that can be administered in much smaller doses to avoid side effects, the male "shot" will not soon replace the female Pill as the single most popular form of temporary contraception in the United States.

Another experimental approach to male contraception is the administration of female hormones. Thus far, both progestins and estrogens have been used with some success, each suppressing sperm production in 70 to 80 percent of the men treated. Like androgens, progestins and estrogens "fool" the pituitary into halting its release of LH and FSH (Steinberger, 1971).

Unfortunately, there are some negative side effects when men take significant doses of female hormones. There is the risk, as yet uncalculated, of genetic damage in cases where spermatogenesis has not been completely suppressed. In addition, high doses of progestins and estrogens, like high doses of androgens, can lead to liver toxicity. Men who take female hormones may also suffer from less dangerous but highly bothersome side effects such as loss of sex drive, increase in weight, night sweats, delayed orgasm, liver pain, nipple pain, painful erections, and, perhaps most embarrassingly, breast enlargement (gynecomastia). To counteract these side effects, researchers have supplemented the female hormones with doses of testosterone either by injection or underskin implants. While this technique alleviates the loss of sex drive and gynecomastia, it has been effective in making men azoospermic in only four out of five cases, a rate that is not acceptable in a contraceptive (Barfield, et al., 1979).

Some researchers interested in readjusting the glandular network for contraception have concentrated on inhibin, a substance that some scientists believe is produced in the seminiferous tubules. Though much remains to be known about its function and its interaction with the pituitary gland, it is believed that the presence of too much inhibin in the bloodstream lowers the pituitary's output of FSH. Thus, if inhibin is injected into the bloodstream, FSH will diminish and, in theory, spermatogenesis should slow or stop entirely. However, the problems with inhibin injections seem even more formidable than those with androgen or female hormone injections. For one thing, inhibin has never been purified or synthesized. For another, excessive levels of inhibin in the bloodstream may lead to liver damage (Djerassi, 1981).

Interfering with Sperm Maturation

When immature sperm are pushed into the convoluted tubing of the epididymis, they cannot swim on their own; sixteen days later, when they emerge at the other end of the epididymis, they are able to swim strongly. Identification of a safe substance that neutralizes sperm during this period of maturation rather than during spermatogenesis would significantly reduce the risk of genetic damage. Unfortunately, research in this area is not extensive and has not progressed very far.

Research on rats has demonstrated that cyproterone acetate is capable of inhibiting sperm maturation in the epididymis, but it also destroys gonadal tissue.

Another chemical, α-chlorhydrin, also inhibits sperm maturation in rats, but it is lethal to monkeys when injected in doses large enough to induce sterility. While it is possible that chemists will one day synthesize a safe, effective contraceptive with a molecular structure similar to cyproterone acetate or α-chlorhydrin, its development and approval for human use remain far in the future (Steinberger, 1971).

Interfering with Sperm Transport

Vasectomy is the most obvious method for interrupting the ejaculation of mature sperm from the reproductive system, but it is not the only possibility. For more than a decade, researchers have been working on various mechanical means to block the movement of sperm through the vas. These means have the advantage of being wholly reversible. One interesting technique is the vas valve, a small device that is sewn into the vas with an on-off switch to block or permit the passage of sperm, depending on the owner's preference. Two kinds of valves have been developed: one must be opened and closed by a urologist through an incision in the scrotum; the other can be opened and closed, in theory at least, by passing a magnet across the scrotum.

In the early 1970s, vas valves were thought to hold great promise as a reversible form of male contraception (Brueschke, et al., 1980). But certain difficulties quickly became apparent. Switching the valves on and off has proven to be quite a problem, particularly in the magnetic types. Valves in the open position do not always allow sperm to flow through freely. Moreover, the surgical implant site is even more prone to leakage and granuloma formation than vasectomy sites. And, like a vasectomy, a closed valve produces pressure building in the epididymis and rete testis that can render a man infertile even after the valve has been switched open. While the concept of a vas valve is clever and appealing, the technology still has a long way to go.

Two other blocking techniques have been tried with limited success: 1) a simple clip surgically placed around the outside of the vas, and 2) a plastic plug or thick thread inside the vas. Aside from causing pressure buildup the clip also seems to damage the inner lining of the vas (lumen), making it difficult or impossible for sperm to pass through when the clip is later removed (Wortman and Piotrow, 1973). Similarly, plastic plugs or threads create pressure, but they may also cause a dilation of the lumen's muscular lining, permitting the sperm to detour freely around the obstruction. In sum, there do not seem to be any simple technological shortcuts in the search for a temporary form of highly effective male birth control.

Sperm Banking

Many people were confident in the early 1970s that vasectomy in combination with sperm banking would become a popular way for a man to take responsibility for birth control. They reasoned that banking sperm, a kind of change-your-mind insurance, would provide an incentive for men considering vasectomy. If the vasectomy could not be reversed by surgical means, artificial insemination with the man's own sperm would still be available as an alternative.

These hopes have not as yet been realized. The freezing techniques currently used at human sperm banks cannot guarantee the viability of sperm. Moreover, it should be pointed out that artificial insemination can be difficult to achieve. On the average, it takes six months of trying for a woman to become pregnant using this method, and for older women it can take considerably longer. Using the techniques associated with the rhythm method of contraception, a woman keeps track of her temperature and the thickness of her cervical mucus to determine when she is ovulating. At this point, she must visit her gynecologist office or the sperm bank, where a physician places a quantity of defrosted ejaculate on or near her cervix. This process can be somewhat unappealing to all but the highly motivated. Should the number of sperm deposits run out before the woman conceives, the couple is then forced to consider using the sperm of an anonymous donor. To date, no researcher has been able to demonstrate that insemination with previously frozen sperm produces pregnancy rates comparable to those resulting from intercourse among normally fertile couples (Amelar and Dubin, 1979).

The inability of sperm banks to guarantee that a vasectomized man can change his mind about not making a child highlights the major theme of this book: a decision for vasectomy should be one that you can live with for the rest of your life. While the improvements in microsurgical reversal techniques will offer more hope for men whose circumstances or feelings change, current success rates run between 50 and 80 percent. Insemination with frozen sperm carries no better odds.

Still it must be acknowledged that hormonal or chemical male birth control is many years away, if it ever appears. Condoms are not completely effective, nor are they carefree to use. Therefore, those men who seriously assume contraceptive responsibility in their relationships must consider vasectomy. Those who are indeed certain that they no longer want to produce offspring in their current or any future circumstances will find vasectomy an uncomplicated, safe means toward this end.

Glossary

Abdomen The skin, fat, and muscle overlying and containing the stomach, intestines and other vital organs.

Abscess A pus-filled pocket of tissue caused by infection.

Anastomosis Surgical joining of two hollow structures, such as the severed ends of the vas in vasectomy reversal.

Androgens Male sex hormones, such as testosterone.

Andrologist A physician who specializes in disorders of the male reproductive system.

Anesthesia Any medical procedure to diminish or eliminate bodily sensation of pain. Local anesthesia, numbing only the area of the scrotum, is usually sufficient for vasectomy; general anesthesia, rendering the patient unconscious, is usually prescribed for reversal.

Antibody Neutralizing agents produced by the body's immune system in response to invasion by a foreign substance or antigen.

Arrhythmia Irregular heart beat.

Artificial insemination Introduction of semen into the uterus using gynecological instruments for the purpose of inducing pregnancy.

Autoimmunity An abnormal allergic response against components of your own body.

Atherosclerosis Hardening and narrowing of the arteries caused by accumulation of fatty substances (plaque) on their inner walls.

Azoospermia Absence of sperm in the ejaculate.

Biopsy Surgical removal of a small piece of tissue for analysis.

Bis-dichlorocetyl A chemical that suppresses sperm production but causes nausea and vomiting when taken with alcoholic beverages.

Castration Surgical removal of the testes.

Cauterization Sealing of small blood vessels or ducts with heat; electrocauterization is commonly used to staunch the bleeding of tiny blood vessels during vasectomy.

Cervix The opening that leads from the vagina to the uterus.

α-chlorhydrin A chemical that suppresses sperm maturation but with some toxic side effects.

Chronic orchialgia Pain in the testicles, sometimes experienced as an aftereffect of vasectomy when fluid accumulates in the sealed vasa.

Condom A male contraceptive sheath made of rubber or animal skin worn over the penis during sexual intercourse.

Contraceptive Any procedure to prevent pregnancy.

Corpus cavernosum Either of paired cylindrical tubes lying on both sides of the corpus spongiosum; they contain channels that become engorged with blood during sexual excitement and are primarily responsible for penile erection.

Corpus spongiosum Spongy tissue surrounding the urethra and head of the penis; it contains channels that engorge with blood during sexual excitement, contributing to erection.

Cryptorchidism Failure of one or both testes to descend into the scrotum.

Culdoscopy Examination of the female pelvic organs through a small surgical opening made in the vagina; also associated with one procedure for tubal ligation.

Cyproterone acetate A synthetic hormone that blocks the action of androgens and suppresses sperm production and maturation.

DES (diethylstilbesterol) A synthetic female sex hormone that has been implicated as a cause of congenital birth defects when taken during pregnancy.

Diaphragm A female contraceptive device; a rubber barrier filled with a spermicidal cream and placed over the cervix.

Dinitropyrrole A toxic chemical that suppresses sperm production.

Ectopic pregnancy Growth of a fertilized egg outside the womb (uterus), usually in a fallopian tube; very dangerous and possibly life-threatening, it may be associated with use of an IUD.

Ejaculate Semen; fluid containing sperm and nutrients that is expelled from the urethra at the time of orgasm.

Ejaculatory duct One of two tubular structures, each formed by the convergence of a vas deferens and a seminal vesicle behind the base of the bladder; here sperm from the vas deferens mix with nutrient fluid from the seminal vesicle.

Electrocautery An electrically heated tweezer or needle used to seal small blood vessels during surgery.

Emission The movement of seminal fluids through the reproductive tract to the bulb of the urethra just prior to ejaculation.

Endocrine Hormonal; describing those bodily organs that produce hormones.

Epididymis The fifteen-foot-long, tightly coiled, thin-walled tube that conducts spermatocytes and fluid from the rete testis to the vas deferens, where they emerge as mature sperm.

Estrogens Female sex hormones.

Eugenics A study dealing with the improvement of hereditary traits by selective breeding.

Fallopian tubes Ducts through which ova (eggs) travel to the uterus; fertilization of eggs by sperm cells occurs in the fallopian tubes.

Fertility The physiological ability to have children.

Fertility clinic A medical facility devoted to the diagnosis and treatment of infertility.

Foam A sperm-killing chemical introduced into the vagina as a contraceptive; marginally effective.

FSH (follicle stimulating hormone) The hormone released with LH by the pituitary gland to stimulate the testes to manufacture sperm.

Fulguration Another word for cauterization.

Gland A bodily organ that produces hormones, enzymes, or other specialized substances.

Glans The head of the penis; in females, the corresponding portion of the clitoris.

Gonads Organs that generate reproductive cells: the testes in men, the ovaries in women.

Gossypol An experimental male anti-fertility drug derived from cottonseed.

Granuloma A ball of inflammation tissue, commonly an aftereffect of vasectomy associated with leakage of sperm from the vas.

Gynecomastia Abnormal enlargement of the male breasts, sometimes resulting from administration of female hormones for contraceptive purposes.

Hematoma An accumulation of blood after surgery; it is a potential aftereffect of vasectomy but more common after reversal.

Hormone The secretion of a specialized gland that influences the function of other bodily cells.

Hypothalamus The gland at the base of the brain that releases LH-RH to control sperm production indirectly through the pituitary gland.

Hysterectomy Removal of the uterus (womb).

Immune complex A foreign substance clumped with neutralizing antibodies produced by the immune system; the foreign substance is then eliminated from the circulatory system.

Immune system The body's defense against invasion by bacteria, viruses, or toxins; after vasectomy, the immune system may identify a man's own sperm as foreign.

Impotence Inability to achieve erection and orgasm.

Indo-carboxylic acid A toxic chemical that suppresses sperm production.

Inhibin A substance possibly produced by the seminiferous tubules that controls secretion of FSH by the pituitary and thus controls sperm production. It has yet to be purified or synthesized.

IUD (intra uterine device) A plastic or metal contraceptive device placed in the uterus.

Laparoscopy Looking inside the abdomen with a special instrument introduced through a small incision; also refers to one method of tubal ligation.

Laparotomy A surgical opening made into the abdomen, associated with tubal ligation.

Leydig cells (interstitial cells) Cells in the testes that manufacture the male sex hormones, primarily testosterone.

LH (luteinizing hormone) A hormone released by the pituitary gland, causing the testes in men and ovaries in women to manufacture sex hormones.

LH-RH (luteinizing hormone-releasing hormone) The hypothalamic hormone that stimulates the pituitary gland to release its hormones, LH and FSH.

Ligate To tie off a blood vessel or tube.

Lumen An opening or channel inside a tubular organ, as in the vasa deferentia or in the fallopian tubes.

Microsurgery Medical operations performed on tiny structures such as nerves, capillaries, or vasa, using surgical microscopes and specialized instruments.

Motility The ability of sperm to swim forward.

Myocardial infarction Heart attack.

Nitrofuran An antibiotic that suppresses sperm production but only when taken in toxic doses.

Norepinephrine An adrenalin-like chemical released by nerve endings in the male reproductive tract to cause ejaculation.

Organ A structure of cells and tissue performing a specialized bodily function.

Orgasm The climax of sexual excitement, culminating in the male with powerful rhythmic contractions throughout the reproductive tract to cause ejaculation.

Ovary The female gonad, where eggs and sex hormones are produced.

Ovum An egg; when fertilized by a sperm, it develops in the uterus until birth.

Pathologist A physician who specializes in the examination and identification of abnormal tissues.

Prostate A gland at the base of the bladder that contributes additional fluid to the ejaculate.

The Pill Orally administered, hormonal contraceptive for women.

Pituitary gland The gland located at the base of the brain that influences many of the body's other glands, including the testes in men and ovaries in women.

Primary sex characteristics The penis and testes in men; the uterus, ovaries, and vagina in women.

Progesterone (progestins) A female sex hormone; important in the natural maintenance of pregnancy, it has also been used for birth control in women and men.

Pulmonary embolism Blockage of a blood vessel supplying the lungs by a blood clot.

Recanalization Formation of new channels through or around a blocked blood vessel, vas deferens, or other tubular structure.

Rete testis A delicate collection of tubes connecting the seminiferous tubules to the epididymis.

Scrotum The sac containing the testicles.

Secondary sex characteristics Traits that are not directly related to reproduction but that typically distinguish men and women: facial hair, pitch of voice, breast development, distribution of muscle and fat, etc.

Semen Secretions of the prostate and seminal vesicles combined with sperm and testicular fluid in the urethra and expelled during ejaculation.

Seminal fluid Semen; the fluid that surrounds and nourishes ejaculated sperm.

Seminal vesicles The paired glands at the base of the bladder that manufacture and secrete the bulk of the seminal fluid.

Seminiferous tubules The network of tubes in the testes where sperm are manufactured.

Sperm (spermatozoa) The male reproductive cells, characterized by a specialized head and tail enabling it to swim through the female reproductive tract.

Spermatocytes The partially differentiated cells in the seminiferous tubules that mature into sperm.

Sphincter A circular muscle that opens and closes a channel of the body, like the urethra.

Sterilization A surgical procedure designed to produce permanent infertility.

Testicular fluid Fluid secreted by the testes that bathes sperm during their maturation.

Testis, testes (testicle, testicles) The male gonads, consisting of seminiferous tubules, which produce sperm, and Leydig cells, which produce male sex hormones.

Testosterone The principal male sex hormone.

Thromboembolism Blockage of a blood vessel by a loose clot floating in the blood stream.

Thrombophlebitis Inflammation of a vein or veins obstructed by blood clot.

Tubal ligation Sterilization of the female by surgical interruption of the fallopian tubes.

Urethra In the male, the tube running from the bladder to the tip of the penis, through which urine and semen are conducted.

Urology A surgical specialty dealing with disorders of the urinary system of both sexes and the reproductive system of men.

Uterus The womb, where a fertilized ovum develops.

Vas deferens The small, fifteen-inch-long tube that conducts sperm and testicular fluid to the ejaculatory ducts.

Vasectomy A male sterilization operation that interrupts both vasa deferentia.

Vasoepididymostomy See vasovasostomy, below.

Vasovasostomy Vasectomy reversal; specifically, surgical reconnection of healthy vas ends at the point where they were severed. If the testicular side of the vas is blocked or damaged, the surgeon performs a vasoepididymostomy, a reconnection that bypasses the blocked or damaged section of epididymis.

References

Chapter 1

Fried, J. J. *Vasectomy: The Truth and Consequences of the Newest Form of Birth Control—Male Sterilization.* New York: Saturday Review Press, 1972.

Gillette, P. J. *The Vasectomy Information Manual.* New York: Outerbridge and Lazard, 1972.

Kasirsky, G. *Vasectomy, Manhood, and Sex.* New York: Springer Publishing, 1972.

Lader, L. *Foolproof Birth Control.* Boston: Beacon Press, 1972.

Wolfers, D. and H. *Vasectomy and Vasectomania.* London: Mayflower Books, Ltd., 1974.

Wylie, E. M. *A Guide to Voluntary Sterilization.* New York: Barnes and Noble, 1973.

Chapter 2

Ewing, L. L. "Testis: Epididymis." In *Urology.* Harrison, et al. Philadelphia: W. B. Saunders and Company, 1978: 134–160.

Hamilton, D. W. and Greep, R. O. "The Male Reproductive System." Volume 5, *Handbook of Physiology.* Washington, D.C.: American Physiological Association, 1975.

Jenkins, A. D., et al. "Physiology of the Male Reproductive System." *Urological Clinics of North America* 5 (1978): 437–450.

Silber, S. J. *The Male: From Infancy to Old Age.* New York: Charles Scribner's Sons, 1981.

Chapter 3

Ager, J. W., et al. "Vasectomy: Who Gets One and Why?" *American Journal of Public Health* 64 (1974): 680–686.

Ferber, A. S., et al. "Men with Vasectomies: A Study of Medical, Sexual, and Psychosocial Changes." *Psychosomatic Medicine* 29 (1967): 354–366.

Howard, G. "Attitudes to Vasectomy." *IPPF Medical Bulletin* 15 (1981): 1–3.

Leavesley, J. H. "A Study of Vasectomized Men and Their Wives." *Australian Family Physician* 9 (1980): 8–10.

Maschhoff, T. A., et al. "Vasectomy: Its Effect Upon Marital Stability." *Journal of Sex Research* 12 (1976): 295–314.

Wolfers, D. and H. *Vasectomy and Vasectomania.* London; Mayflower Books, Ltd., 1974.

Chapter 4

Bedford, J. M. and Zelikovsky, G. "Viability of Spermatozoa in the Human Ejaculate After Vasectomy." *Fertility and Sterility* 32 (1979): 546–550.

Esho, J. O. and Cass, A. S. "Recanalization Rate Following Methods of Vasectomy Using Interposition of Fascial Sheath of Vas Deferens." *Journal of Urology* 120 (1978): 178–179.

Freund, M. and Davis, J. E. "Disappearance Rate of Spermatozoa from the Ejaculate Following Vasectomy." *Fertility and Sterility* 20 (1969): 163–170.

Hackett, R. E. and Waterhouse, K. "Vasectomy: Reviewed." *American Journal of Obstetrics and Gynecology* 116 (1973): 438–455.

Leader, A. J., et al. "Complications of 2,711 Vasectomies." *Journal of Urology* 111 (1974): 365–369.

Moss, W. M. "Sutureless Vasectomy, an Improved Technique: 1300 Cases Performed Without Failure." *Fertility and Sterility* 27 (1974): 1040–1045.

Schmidt, S. S. "Spermatic Granuloma: An Often Painful Lesion." *Fertility and Sterility* 31 (1979): 178–181.

Shapiro, E. I. and Silber, S. J. "Open-Ended Vasectomy, Sperm Granuloma, and Postvasectomy Orchialgia." *Fertility and Sterility* 32 (1979): 546–550.

Zeigler, F. J., et al. "Psychosocial Response to Vasectomy." *Archives of General Psychiatry* 21 (1969): 46–54.

Chapter 5

Barglow, P. "Pseudocyesis and Psychiatric Sequelae of Sterilization." *Archives of General Psychiatry* 11 (1964): 571–580.

Bloom, L. J. and Houston, B. K. "The Psychological Effects of Vasectomy for American Men." *Journal of Genetic Psychology* 128 (1976): 173–182.

Brown, R. A., and Magarick, R. H. "Psychologic Effects of Vasectomy in Voluntarily Childless Men." *Urology* 14 (1979): 55–58.

Denniston, G. C. "The Effects of Vasectomy on Childless Men." *Journal of Reproductive Medicine* 21 (1978): 151–152.

Doty, F. O. "Emotional Aspects of Vasectomy: A Review." *Journal of Reproductive Medicine* 10 (1973): 156–161.

Ferber, A. S., et al. "Men with Vasectomies: A Study of Medical, Sexual, and Psychosocial Changes." *Psychosomatic Medicine* 29 (1967): 354–366.

Fitzgerald, J. A. "The Female Response to Vas Ligation." *Medical Insight* (January 1972): 22–26.

Hamersma, R. J., et al. "Psychological Dynamics and Self-Perceptions of Vasectomy Candidates." *Perceptual and Motor Skills* 40 (1975): 1004–1006.

Horenstein, D. and Houston, B. K. "Effects of Vasectomy on Postoperative Psychological Adjustment and Self-Concept." *Journal of Psychology* 89 (1975): 167–173.

Howard, G. "Attitudes to Vasectomy." *IPPF Medical Bulletin* 15 (1981): 1–3.

Janke, L. D. and Weist, W. M. "Psychosocial and Medical Effects of Vasectomy in a Sample of Health Plan Subscribers." *International Journal of Psychiatry in Medicine* 7 (1976): 17–34.

Leavesley, J. H. "A Study of Vasectomized Men and Their Wives." *Australian Family Physician* 9 (1980): 8–10.

Lieberman, R. G., et al. "Vasectomy for the Single, Childless Man." *Journal of Family Practice* 8 (1979): 181–184.

Maschhoff, T. A., et al. "Vasectomy: Its Effect Upon Marital Stability." *Journal of Sex Research* 12 (1976): 295–314.

Vaughn, R. L. "Behavioral Response to Vasectomy." *Archives of General Psychiatry* 36 (1979): 815–821.

Weist, W. M. and Janke, L. D. "A Methodological Critique of Research on Psychological Effects of Vasectomy." *Psychosomatic Medicine* 36 (1974): 438–449.

Wolfers, H. "Psychological Aspects of Vasectomy." *British Medical Journal* 4 (1970): 297–300.

Zeigler, F. J., et al. "Psychosocial Response to Vasectomy." *Archives of General Psychiatry* 21 (1969): 46–54.

Zeigler, F. J. "Male Sterilization." *Sexual Behavior* (July 1971): 71–73.

Chapter 6

Alexander, N. J. and Henderson, D. J. "Vasectomy: Consequences of Autoimmunity to Sperm Antigens." *Fertility and Sterility* 32 (1979): 253–260.

Bullock, J. Y., et al. "Autoantibodies Following Vasectomy." *Journal of Urology* 118 (1977): 602–603.

Clarkson, T. B. and Alexander, N. J. "Long-Term Vasectomy: Effects on the Occurrence and Extent of Atherosclerosis in Rhesus Monkeys." *Journal of Clinical Investigation* 65 (1980): 15–25.

Editorial. "Safety of Vasectomy." *The Lancet* (November 17, 1979): 1057–1058.

Editorial. "Vasectomy—A Note of Concern: Reprise." *Journal of the American Medical Association* 245 (1981): 2333.

Lepow, I. H. and Crozier, R., eds. *Immunologic and Pathophysiologic Effects in Animals and Man.* New York: Academic Press, 1979.

Linnet, L., et al. "Association Between Failure to Impregnate After Vasovasostomy and Sperm Agglutinins in Semen." *The Lancet* (January 17, 1981): 117–119.

Petitti, D. B., et al. "Physiologic Measures in Men with and without Vasectomies." *Fertility and Sterility* 37 (1982): 438–440.

Richards, I. S. "Current Status of Endocrinologic Effects of Vasectomy." *Urology* 18 (1981): 1–6.

Roberts, H. J. *Is Vasectomy Safe?* West Palm Beach: Sunshine Academic Press, 1979.

Silber, S. J. "Sperm Granuloma and Reversibility of Vasectomy." *The Lancet* (September 17, 1977): 588–589.

Smith, M. S. and Paulson, D. F. "The Physiologic Consequences of Vas Ligation." *Urological Survey* 30 (1980): 31–33.

Verheught, F. W., et al. "Vasectomy and Cholesterol." *New England Journal of Medicine* (August 20, 1981): 462.

Wallace, R. B., et al. "Vasectomy and Coronary Disease in Men Less Than 50 Years Old: Absence of Association." *Journal of Urology* 126 (1981): 182–184.

Walker, A. M., et al. "Hospitalization Rates in Vasectomized Men." *Journal of the American Medical Association* 245 (1981a): 2315–2317.

―――――. "Vasectomy and Non-Fatal Myocardial Infarction." *The Lancet* (January 3, 1981b): 13–15.

Chapter 7

Barglow, P. "Pseudocyesis and Psychiatric Sequelae of Sterilization." *Archives of General Psychiatry* 11 (1964): 571–580.

Ford, K. "Contraceptive Efficacy Among Married Women 15–44 Years of Age in the United States, 1970–73." *Advancedata* 26 (1978): 1–3.

Free, M., and Alexander, N. J. "Male Contraception Without Prescription: A Re-Evaluation of the Condom and Coitus Interruptus." *Public Health Reports* 91 (1976): 437–445.

Hatcher, R. A., et al. *Contraceptive Technology, 1976–1977.* New York: Irvington Publishers, 1976.

Howard, G. "Attitudes to Vasectomy." *IPPF Medical Bulletin* 15 (1981): 1–3.

Jick, H., et al. "Oral Contraceptives and Nonfatal Myocardial Infarction." *Journal of the American Medical Association* 239 (1978): 1403–1404.

Layde, P. M., et al. "Further Analyses of Mortality in Oral Contraceptive Users." *Lancet* (March 7, 1981): 541–546.

McCann, M. F., and Kessel, E. "International Experience with Laparoscopic Sterilization: Follow-up of 8500 Women." *Advances in Planned Parenthood* 12 (1978): 199–211.

Mumford, S. D., and Bhiwandiwala, P. R. "Tubal Ring Sterilization: Experience with 10,086 Cases." *Obstetrics and Gynecology* 57 (1981): 150–157.

Roberts, H. J. *Is Vasectomy Safe?* West Palm Beach: Sunshine Academic Press, 1979.

Rosenfield, A. "Oral and Intrauterine Contraception: A 1978 Risk Assessment." *American Journal of Obstetrics and Gynecology* 132 (1978): 92–106.

Stadel, B. "Oral Contraceptives and Cardiovascular Disease (First of Two Parts)." *New England Journal of Medicine* 305 (1981): 612–618.

————. "Oral Contraceptives and Cardiovascular Disease (Second of Two Parts)." *New England Journal of Medicine* 305 (1981): 672–677.

Tucker, Tarvez. *Birth Control.* New York: Dell Publishing, 1981.

Vessey, M. "Female Hormones and Vascular Disease—An Epidemiological Overview." *British Journal of Family Planning—Supplement* 6 (1980): 1–12.

Vessey, M., et al. "A Long-Term Follow-Up Study of Women Using Different Methods of Contraception—An Interim Report." *Journal of Biosocial Science* 8 (1976): 373–427.

————. "Mortality in Oral Contraceptive Users." *Lancet* (March 7, 1981): 549–550.

Chapter 8

Editorial. "Vasectomy Reversal." *The Lancet* 1 (September 20, 1980): 625–626.

Fenster, H. and McLoughlin, M. G. "Vasovasostomy—Microscopic versus Macroscopic Techniques." *Archives of Andrology* 7 (1981): 201–204.

Fernandes, M., Shah, K. N., and Draper, J. W. "Vasovasostomy: Improved Microsurgical Technique." *Journal of Urology* 100 (1968): 763–766.

Hampel, N., et al. "Microsurgical Anastomosis of Vas Deferens: An Experimental Study in the Rat." *Investigative Urology* 15 (1978): 395–396.

Lee, L. and McLoughlin, M. G. "Vasovasostomy: A Comparison of Macroscopic and Microscopic Techniques at One Institution." *Fertility and Sterility* 33 (1980): 54–55.

Linnet, L., Hjort, T., and Fogh-Anderson, P. "Association Between Failure to Impregnate After Vasovasostomy and Sperm Agglutinins in Semen." *The Lancet* (January 17, 1981): 117–119.

Owen, E. R. "Microsurgical Vasovasostomy: A Reliable Vasectomy Reversal." *Australia and New Zealand Journal of Surgery* 47 (1977): 305–309.

Silber, S. J. "Microscopic Vasectomy Reversal." *Fertility and Sterility* 28 (1977a): 1191–1202.

————. "Sperm Granuloma and Reversibility of Vasectomy." *The Lancet* (September 17, 1977b): 588–589.

————. "Microscopic Vasoepididymostomy: Specific Microanastomosis to the Epididymal Tubule." *Fertility and Sterility* 30 (1978a): 565–570.

————. "Vasectomy and Vasectomy Reversal." *Fertility and Sterility* 29 (1978b): 125–140.

Thomas, A. J., Jr., et al. "Vasovasostomy: Evaluation of Four Surgical Techniques." *Fertility and Sterility* 32 (1979): 324–328.

Chapter 9

Decker, A., and Loebl, S. *Why Can't We Have a Baby? An Authority Looks at the Causes and Cures of Childlessness.* New York: Warner Books, 1979.

Fenton, J. A. and Lifchez, A. S., *The Fertility Handbook.* New York: Clarkson N. Potter, Inc., 1980.

Harrison, M. *Infertility: A Guide for Couples.* Boston: Houghton Mifflin Company, 1977.

Menning, B. E. *Infertility: A Guide for the Childless Couple.* Riverside, CA: NACAC, 1980.

Silber, S. J. *How to Get Pregnant.* New York: Charles Scribner's Sons, 1980.

Chapter 10

Amelar, R. D. and Dubin, L. "Frozen Semen—A Poor Form of Fertility Insurance." *Urology* 14 (1979): 53–54.

Barfield, A., et al. "Pregnancies Associated with Sperm Concentrations Below 10 Million per Milliliter in Clinical Studies of a Potential Male Contraceptive Method, Monthly Depot Medroxyprogesterone and Testosterone Esters. *Contraception* 20 (1979): 121–127.

Beck, W. W., and Silverstein, I. "Variable Motility Recovery of Spermatozoa Following Freeze Preservation." *Fertility and Sterility* 26 (1975): 863–867.

Brueschke, E. E., et al. "Development of a Reversible Vas Deferens Occlusive Device. VII. Physical and Microscopic Observations After Long-Term Implantation of Flexible Prosthetic Devices." *Fertility and Sterility* 33 (1980): 167–178.

Djerassi, C. *The Politics of Contraception.* San Francisco: W. H. Freeman and Company, 1981.

Lardner, T. S. "Bioengineering Aspects of Reproduction and Contraceptive Development." In *Frontiers of Reproduction and Fertility Control.* R. O. Greep and M. S. Koblinsky, eds. Cambridge: MIT Press, 1977.

Reading, A. E., et al. "A Survey of Attitudes Towards Permanent Contraceptive Methods." *Journal of Biosocial Science* 12 (1980): 383–392.

Shearer, S. B. "Current Efforts to Develop Male Hormonal Contraception." *Studies in Family Planning* 9 (1978): 229–231.

Steinberger, E. "Hormonal Control of Mammalian Spermatogenesis." *Physiological Review* 51 (1971): 1–22.

Wortman, J. and Piotrow, P. T. "Vasectomy—Old and New Techniques." *Population Reports* Series D, Number 1 (1973).

List of
Counseling Services

The following is a partial list of marriage and family counselors and counseling centers specializing in helping individuals and couples resolve such issues as family planning, contraceptive practices, and sterilization decision making. If you live in an area not served by one of these counselors or counseling centers and would like a referral to a family counselor in your area, you may write or call:

C. Ray Fowler, Ph.D., Executive Director
American Association for Marriage and Family
    Therapy
924 W. Ninth
Upland, CA 91786
(714) 981-0888

California

Robert J. Green, Ph.D.
The Redwood Center for
    Family and Individual
    Therapy
2372 Ellsworth Street
Berkeley, CA 94704

Walter Kempler, M.D.
The Kempler Institute
P.O. Box 1692
Mesa, CA 92626

Alan F. Leveton, M.D.
Family Therapy Center
    Association
3529 Sacramento Street
San Francisco, CA 94118

Larry Allman, Ph.D.
Los Angeles Family Institute
1315 Westwood Boulevard
Los Angeles, CA 90024

District of Columbia
Marguerite and Julius Fogel,
    M.D.
3948 Brandywine
Washington, DC 20008

Illinois
Charles and Jeannette Kramer
Family Institute of Chicago
10 E. Huron Street
Chicago, IL 60611

Anne Seiden, M.D.
Cook County Hospital
1835 W. Harrison
Chicago, IL 60612

Maryland
Jane and Vincent Sweeny, M.D.
Center for the Study of Human
    Systems
8604 Jones Mill Road
Chevy Chase, MD 20015

Massachusetts
Bunny and Fred Duhl, M.D.
Boston Family Institute
251 Harvard Street
Brookline, MA 02146

Carol Nadelson, M.D.
30 Amory Street
Brookline, MA 02146

Derek Polonsky, M.D.
Tufts New England Medical
    Center
171 Harrison Avenue
Boston, MA 02111

Norman Paul, M.D.
720 Harrison Avenue
Boston, MA 02118

Michigan
Dr. Peter Martin
900 Wall Street
Ann Arbor, MI 48118

New York
Clifford Sager, M.D.
35 E. 75th Street
New York, NY 10021

Ira Glick, M.D.
Family Therapy Project
525 E. 68th Street
New York, NY 10021

Dorothy Strauss, Ph.D.
Robert Dickes, M.D.
Downstate Medical Center
450 Clarkson Avenue
Brooklyn, NY 11203

Association for Voluntary
    Sterilization
122 E. 42nd St.
New York, NY 10168

Ohio
Steve Levine, M.D.
2035 Abington Road
Cleveland, OH 44106

Pennsylvania

Ilda V. Ficher
Department of Mental Health
  Science
Hahnemann Medical College
230 N. Broad Street
Philadelphia, PA 19102

Ellen Berman, M.D.
Marriage Council of
  Philadelphia
4025 Chestnut Street
Philadelphia, PA 19104

Ellen Frank, MSW
Carol Anderson, MSW
Department of Psychology
University of Pittsburgh
3811 O'Hara Street
Pittsburgh, PA 15260

South Carolina

Oliver Bjornsten, M.D.
University of South Carolina
  Medical Center
80 Barre Street
Charleston, SC 29401

Texas

Alberto Serrano, M.D.
Bexar County Mental Health
  Center
4502 Medical Drive
San Antonio, TX 78284

Coping with Infertility

In Chapter 9, we identified some of the ways in which infertility after a reversal attempt can impose stress and communication difficulties in a relationship. For help in dealing with these problems, contact any of the individuals listed above; the organizations listed below can give you a referral to a counselor in your area.

The American Fertility
  Foundation
1608 Thirteenth Avenue South
Birmingham, AL 35205
(205) 933-7222

Resolve, Inc.
P.O. Box 474
Belmont, MA 02178
(617) 484-2424

Barren Foundation
6 East Monroe Street
Chicago, IL 60603
(312) 751-4038

New York Fertility Research
  Foundation, Inc.
123 East 89th Street
New York, NY 10028
(212) 876-9300

Index

Page numbers in *italics* refer to figures or tables.

About the Authors

Marc Goldstein, M.D., is the Director of the Male Repro-
duction and Urologic Microsurgery Unit at New York
Hospital-Cornell Medical Center, Division of Urology,
and an Associate Physician at Rockefeller University
Hospital. He is also a Staff Scientist at the Center for
Biomedical Research, Population Council.

Michael Feldberg, Ph.D., is a Research Associate at the
center for Applied Social Science, Boston University
and is a family therapist-in-training at the Boston
Family Institute. He has undergone both the vasectomy
and reversal operations.

The Vasectomy Book was composed in Aster
by Auto-Graphics, Inc., Monterey Park, California.